SECRETS to Preventing Back and Neck Pain

----

60 WAYS TO PROTECT <u>YOUR</u> SPINE

Josh Zumstein, D.C., M.S.

For information, contact The Back Safety and Wellness Consultants at www.backsafetyandwellness.com

FIRST EDITION

Cover design by Amber Dunk

Cover image © iStockphoto

Edited by Bruce Zumstein and Tom Golden

Library of Congress Cataloging-in-Publication Data has been applied for.

ISBN 978-0-9853121-0-7 (Bound)
ISBN 978-0-9853121-1-4 (E-book)

DISCLAIMER

The purpose of this book is to educate and inform. The author and The Back Safety and Wellness Consultants shall not be held liable or responsible for any damage or loss caused or alleged to be caused, indirectly or directly, by the contents of this book. If you do not choose to abide by the aforementioned, you may return this book for a full refund, with proof of purchase, and within 60 days of purchase, to the site where you purchased it.

To:

My parents, and the 5.6 billion people that will suffer back pain
at some point in their lives

SECRETS to Preventing Back and Neck Pain

----

60 WAYS TO PROTECT <u>YOUR</u> SPINE

TABLE OF CONTENTS

INTRODUCTION

Think of ten people. It doesn't matter their age, gender, race, level of fitness, level of education, profession, or if they are employed. Eight of those ten people will experience back pain at some point in their lives (2). Back pain affects whomever it wants. Low back problems alone cause employees to miss 93 million workdays a year and accrue over $5 billion in health care costs annually (4). Imagine what those numbers would be if they included the neck or upper back!

Upon learning these staggering statistics, I was curious. I've wondered: in the state where I reside, how many workman's compensation injuries result from back injuries? According to the state's Industrial Commission Report, there are over 200,000 work-related incidents, and the back is the most frequently injured body part. This same report says that my home state has paid $2.7 billion in 2007 for workman's compensation benefit payments, and the payouts have increased annually since 1999 (1). The state is paying significant amounts of money for a problem that is primarily preventable! Eighty-five percent of back injuries are of unknown etiology, or in layman's terms—from repetitive misuse (2). Education can prevent repetitive misuse injuries. Furthermore, I've looked at states surrounding my home state, and these adjacent states (3, 5) report either the low back or the combination of back, neck, and trunk injuries as the number one source for their workman's comp claims. At a time when the federal government wants to increase the national debt ceiling and states are out of money, health care costs need to be minimized. Preventing back pain is a great start.

As a health care practitioner, I know firsthand that our industry treats injuries well, but is poor at preventing them. My goal is for every person to know how to prevent back injuries and protect his or her back at home and work. I've written this book after practicing in clinic and talking with my patients. Almost every patient has asked me the same thing: why does my back hurt, and how can I make it feel better. I've spent countless hours researching the best answers to those questions and you will find them in this book.

The purpose of this book is to teach you how to prevent back injuries and protect your back without unnecessary expense or the cost of a health care practitioner. The exercises I recommend are designed for everyone, not just the fit athlete. However, I provide a way to advance the exercises, if needed. This book is not filled with complicated medical text that only doctors can understand. It is for you and me. There are few, if any, books available to the layperson that teach back safety and injury prevention. Previously, only health care practitioners have had access to this information. Not anymore. This book lets the secrets out of the bag, or "doctor's bag," I should say.

It is no wonder why myriad back problems exist—people don't know any different! After reading this book, feel confident you will know how to protect your back from injury, reduce your risk of injury, and prevent any current problem from becoming worse.

HOW TO USE THIS BOOK

This book is divided into three sections: lifestyle, tasks, and exercises. "Lifestyle" teaches common, everyday activities, while "tasks" explains how to perform common tasks properly. The "exercises" section discusses the correct way to perform exercises that are most commonly done incorrectly, and how to strengthen spine-stabilizing muscles.

After each of the 60 "secrets," you'll see "RELATED NUMBERS" at the bottom of the page. These "related numbers" identify other "secrets" mentioned in the book that are similar to the "secret" you just read. You may refer to these other secrets mentioned in the related numbers to advance your understanding. Do not confuse the "related numbers" at the bottom of the page with the cited references appearing in parentheses within the text. The cited references refer to the numbered references found at the end of this introduction (see below) and each chapter.

I recommend using certain products for a handful of the 60 "secrets." It may be difficult to locate these products, so for your convenience I've listed my website, **www.backsafetyandwellness.com**, as a place to purchase these exact products.

Now, it's time for you to enjoy the benefits of your investment and get your life back!

REFERENCES

1. Illinois Workers' Compensation Commission 2009 Report. PDF file.
2. Liebenson, Craig. *Rehabilitation of the Spine: A Practitioners Manual.* 2nd ed. Baltimore: Lippincott, 2007. Print.
3. Missouri Department of Workman's Compensation 2009 Annual Report. PDF File.
4. Oz, Mehmet, M.D. "Dr. Oz." Time Magazine 7 Mar. 2011: 90. Print.
5. Wisconsin Workers' Compensation Hygiene Lab Annual Reports on Injury and Illness Claims. Annual Report 2008. PDF File.

CHAPTER 1: LIFESTYLE

1. AVOID FLEXION OF THE SPINE

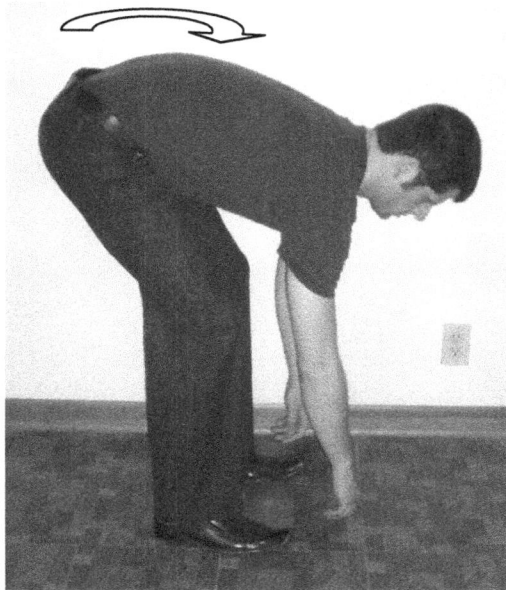

FIGURE 1 – AVOID THIS "C-SHAPE"

What is flexion of the spine? Flexion, also known as bending, occurs when you bend forward to pick up an object off the floor, tie your shoes, etc. The action of repeatedly fully bending the spine is a risk factor for low back disorders and causes disc herniations (bulging discs) in the spine. In addition, bending your spine for a prolonged period of time will damage your back. Note the "C-shaped" hump in the low back of FIGURE 1. This "C-shaped" hump indicates flexion of the spine and incorrect bending. Whenever you see this "C-shape" in the low back, you are bending incorrectly!

It is best to avoid repeated and prolonged flexion of the spine. It is also important to understand that every time you bend forward, you must extend your back to get up again. This act of straightening your back after bending forward is called extension. Cycles of bending forward and coming back up cause low back problems. Flexion and extension can harm your back without lifting an object. It is simply the act of flexing and extending that is inherently bad. Eliminating flexion (bending) of the spine is critical to protecting your back. After reading this book, you'll learn alternatives to flexing and extending your back so you can save your spine (11,12).

RELATED NUMBERS: 2, 32-35

2. AVOID REPEATED FLEXION/EXTENSION

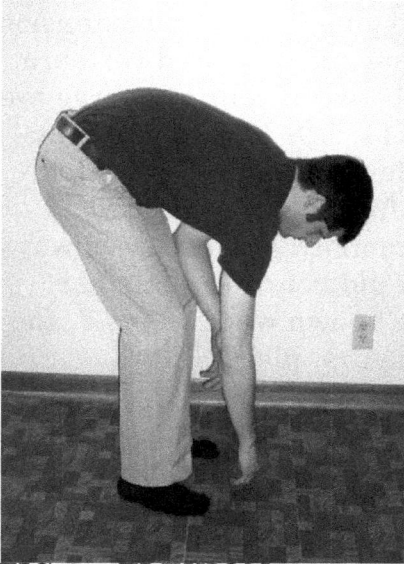
FIG.2 – FLEXION

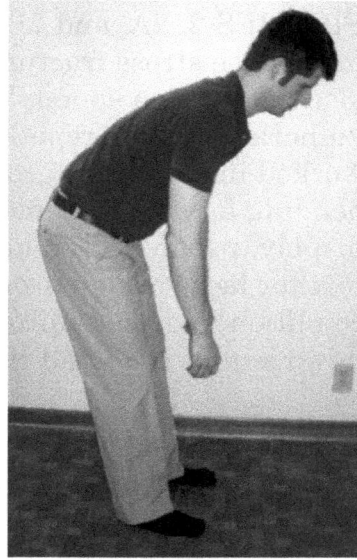
FIG.2A – EXTENSION

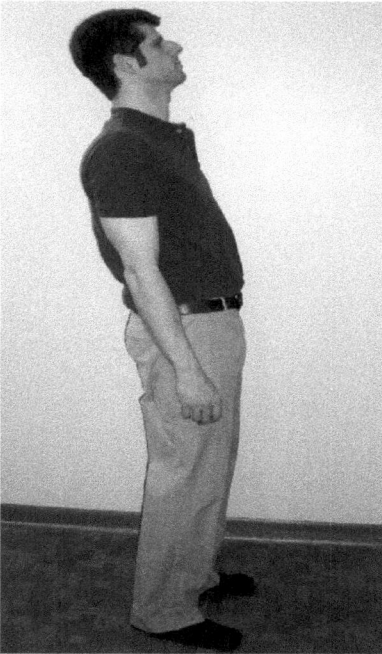
FIG.2B – EXTENSION

Repeatedly bending forward and subsequently straightening your spine is known as flexion and extension (See FIGURES 2, 2A, and 2B). Cyclic full spine flexion and extension may cause stress fractures in the spine and displaced vertebra, also known as a spondylo. The discs between your vertebrae are vulnerable to this repetition as well (11, 12). A patient of mine worked in a deli at a grocery store. Her job required repeatedly bending forward to remove products from the refrigerated display, which caused her spinal discomfort. We discussed ways to alter her work environment so she did not exacerbate her condition and she improved. Had she known what to avoid, she never would have had the issue in the first place.

RELATED NUMBERS: 1, 32-35

3. DON'T BEND AFTER SLEEPING

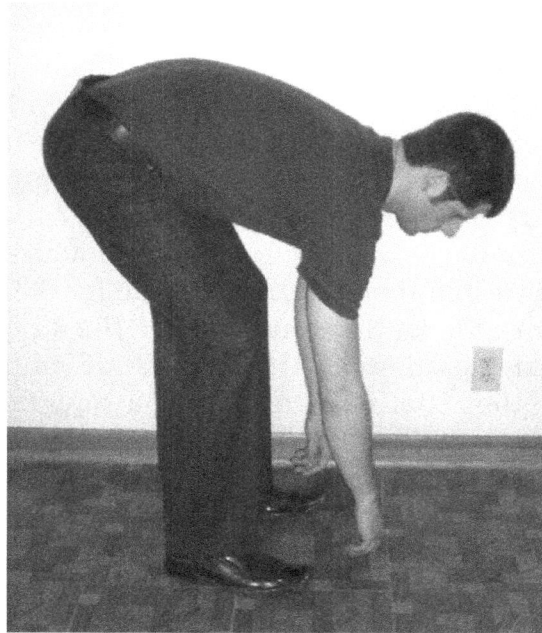

FIGURE 3 – AVOID THIS TECHNIQUE

The spine consists of discs in between each vertebra, which allow for movement and cushion. These discs are primarily made of fluid, which is lost during the day and reabsorbed while you sleep, in a process known as *disc imbibition*. In fact, we lose up to 19 mm of height each day from the loss of disc fluid! After lying down for 2-3 hours, the discs reabsorb their lost fluid and are at full size. When they are full size, the potential stresses placed on the discs are increased by 300%. As a result, it is imperative not to flex/bend your spine (FIGURE 3) for one hour after you have rested for at least 2-3 hours (11, 12). If you must bend during this time, try squatting or hip rotation (secrets #33 and #34). Avoiding flexion of the spine after 2-3 hours of sleep is a great way to protect your back. Please understand, that I'm not saying you can't bend during these aforementioned times, I'm saying it is especially important that you bend the CORRECT way, which you will learn.

RELATED NUMBERS: 1,4, 27-31, 33-35

4.   DON'T BEND AFTER SITTING 20 MINUTES

The muscles, discs, and ligaments of the spine adapt to sustained positions. For example, after 20 minutes of sitting, the soft tissues of your body retain the flexed (bent), seated position. So, if you were to flex your spine, which is the incorrect way to bend after sitting for 20 minutes, you would put your spine at risk for injury (FIGURE 3). This concept is called "*spinal memory*." Similarly to lying down for 2-3 hours, I do not recommend flexing (bending) your spine for 30 minutes after you've sat for at least 20 minutes. Give the spine time to "forget" the previously adapted position (11, 12). If you must bend your back within that 30 minute time period, squat or use hip rotation (secrets #33 and 34).

RELATED NUMBERS: 1,3, 6-11, 32-35

5. STEP FORWARD TO REACH

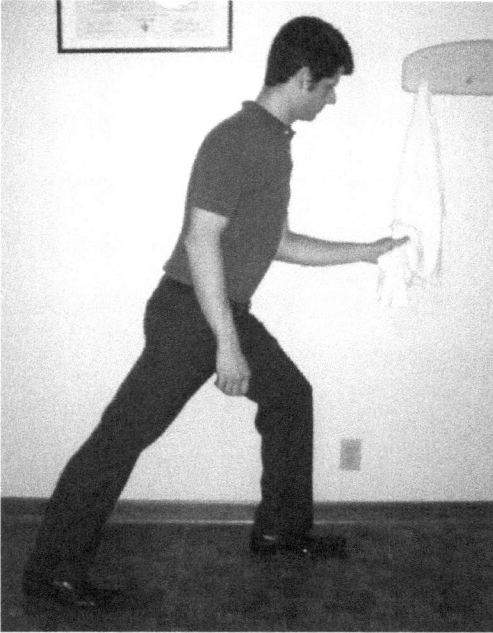

FIGURE 5 – GOOD

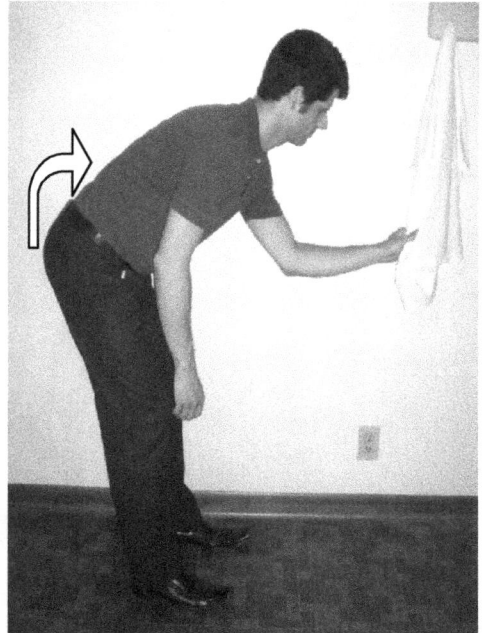

FIGURE 5A – BAD

An alternative to flexing/bending your back to reach for an object is to step forward. Keep your spine neutral as you step forward (FIGURE 5) to reach for an object to prevent the use of your spine and protect your back (11). Notice the difference between the two photos. In FIGURE 5, the back is neutral (straight), whereas FIGURE 5A demonstrates a flexed back with that nasty "C-shape" that you want to avoid. Recall that cyclic full spine flexion and extension causes back injuries. Stepping forward to reach is an alternative to flexion and extension of the spine.

RELATED NUMBERS: 1-2

6. SIT PROPERLY

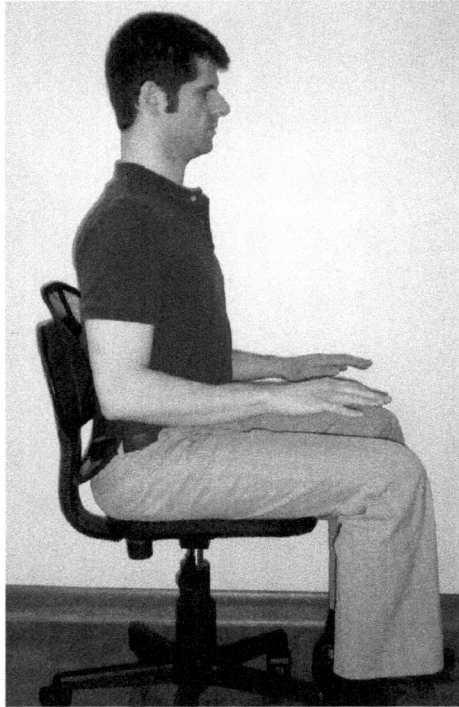

FIGURE 6 – GOOD TECHNIQUE

The perfect seated position is one that changes. There is no ideal seated position, because it is the act of sitting that is inherently bad. However, let's say you are required to sit for an hour without moving, while working at a computer. In this situation, there is a way to sit that will do the least amount of harm. To clarify, this advice applies to the person who is not able to stand up and stretch for a rest break (secret #10) OR use an ergonomic chair (secret #8). In this instance, the perfect seated position involves having perfect posture (FIGURE 6). Note the head is balanced in neutral position, meaning it's not too far forward or backward. Neutral position involves a slight chin tuck—almost as if you are on the verge of a double-chin, but not as extreme. The back is erect with the shoulders pulled back, hips are moved backward at 90 degrees (avoiding the "C-shaped" hump in the low back), feet are flat on the floor, shoulders are not shrugged, elbows are at 90 degrees and wrists are not bent

(11, 12). If you are not working at a computer, you need not worry about your elbows and wrists. However, don't shrug your shoulders. Note that I am using a (secret #7) lumbar support to induce extension into my low back and prevent slouching.

A person, who cannot change positions or take a stretch break while sitting, may sit on a "vestibular disc." A vestibular disc as an inflatable, 1-2 inch thick cushion that health care practitioners typically use to restore balance. These special "cushions" force you to keep a dynamic seated position. I've witnessed numerous patients in clinic improve their back pain and discomfort after sitting on vestibular discs. Because I've personally seen their benefit, I'm comfortable recommending them for you. I suggest sitting on one (with the smooth surface facing up) for 20-30 minutes out of an hour for the first week or two of use. If you don't experience discomfort after 20-30 minutes out of the hour, try sitting on the disc for the entire hour. I don't recommend sitting on an exercise ball, as research does exist stating the disadvantages of using an exercise ball DO NOT exceed the advantages (2, 9, 13).

Visit my website, **www.backsafetyandwellness.com/products**, to find the specific vestibular discs I recommend.

RELATED NUMBERS: 1, 7-11, 24, 32

7. USE A LUMBAR SUPPORT

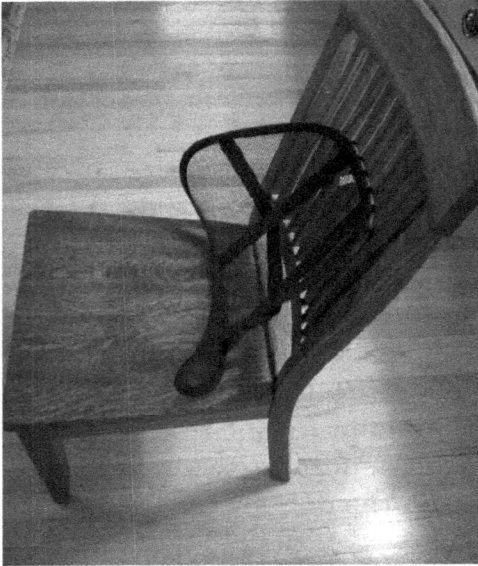

FIGURE 7 – CHAIR   FIGURE 7A – CAR

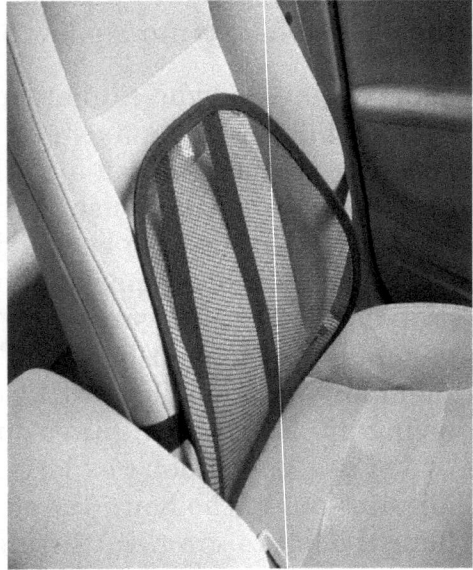

Sitting is harmful. Most seated surfaces are designed for comfort, but fail to provide proper support for the back. This lack of support can cause disc herniations, also known as bulging discs (14). It is this repetitive misuse that leads to 85% of low back injuries (11). To prevent injury from sitting improperly, use a lumbar support. Lumbar supports are inexpensive and may be transferred to different seated areas (FIGURE 7 and 7A). Most cars are equipped with an inherent lumbar support. However, I believe an accessory lumbar support is more efficient. Make sure you are using it correctly. If used correctly, your low back will not have a "C-shaped" hump while you use the support, and you won't slouch. The lumbar support should not come up higher than the bottom of your shoulder blade (8, 14).

Go to **www.backsafetyandwellness.com/products** to find the exact lumbar support that I recommend.

RELATED NUMBERS: 1, 6, 11, 19

8.   USE AN ERGONOMIC CHAIR

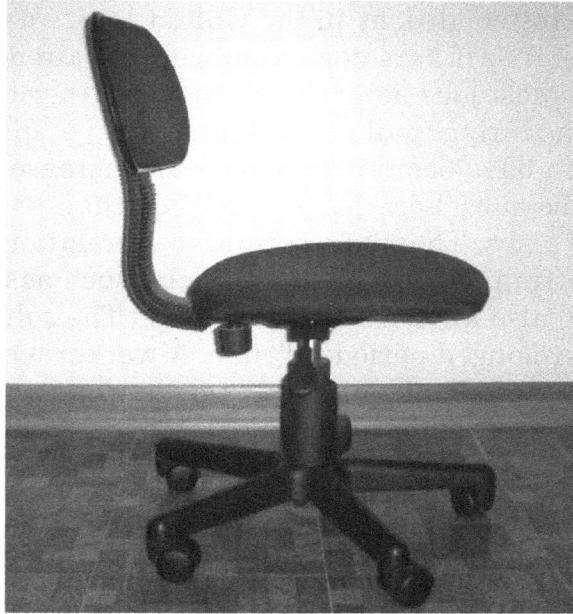

FIGURE 8 – BASIC ERGONOMIC CHAIR

The most ideal seated position is one that changes. An ergonomic chair allows you to adopt different seated positions more easily than regular chairs. Be sure the ergonomic chair allows seat adjustments forward, backward, and side-to-side. It needs to have an adjustable seat height and wheels. If it has arms (which is not necessary), be sure the arms are height adjustable. Do not place your shoulders in a shrugged position. It is equally important that the chair allows for a slight recline. In fact, 95-105 degrees is the ideal seat back position, not 90 degrees (8, 11, 12). The ergonomic chair in FIGURE 8 is a basic ergonomic chair. I featured this chair to show that it is not necessary to spend a fortune on an ergonomic chair to reap its benefits.

Visit my website, **www.backsafetyandwellness.com/products** to find links to companies that sell appropriate ergonomic chairs.

RELATED NUMBERS: 6-7, 9-11

9. DON'T SIT TOO LONG

Working conditions in the United States demand less physically of its workers now, than were required of its workers in the past. Most jobs now involve sitting rather than laborious tasks such as lifting, pulling, pushing, etc., yet disability claims for back pain have been increasing. This increase occurs because sitting can be more harmful to your body than physically demanding tasks. There is a definitive correlation between excessive sitting and low back disorders, such as disc herniations, also known as bulging discs. The solution is to avoid sitting for prolonged periods of time. A worker who sits longer than 50 minutes should stand up, take a walk, or stretch (12), though I recommend he shouldn't sit longer than 20-30 minutes due to the effects of spinal memory (secret #4).

This information is particularly useful to any athlete, such as a baseball or basketball player, who sits for 20 minutes or longer before performing. Because sitting places your back in a stressful position, athletes are at a higher risk for injury if they immediately perform their athletic tasks after sitting for 20-30 minutes or longer. If an athlete must sit for an extended period of time before playing, he/she must remember to sit with proper posture, take stretch breaks, or use a vestibular disc (see secret #6, or visit my website, **www.backsafetyandwellness.com/products**).

RELATED NUMBERS: 6-8, 10-11, 24, 32

10. STRETCH EVERY 20-30 MINUTES

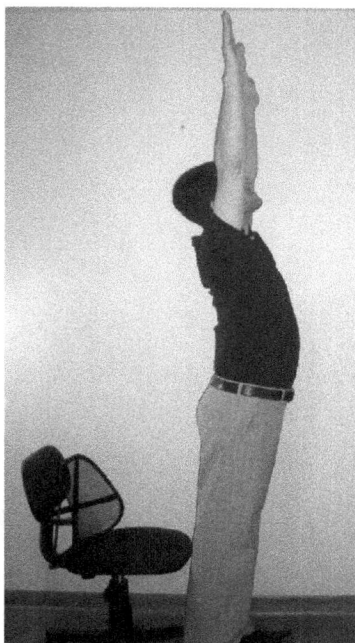

FIGURE 10 – REACH

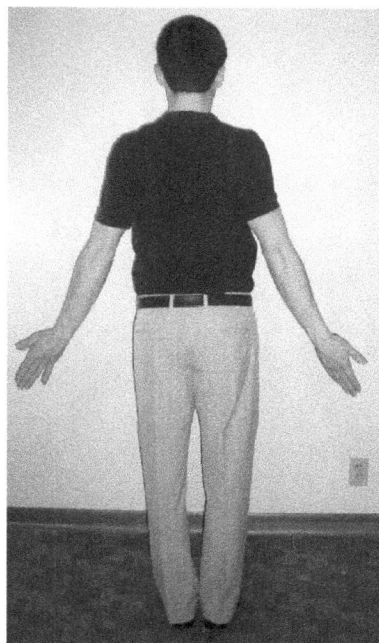

FIGURE 10A – SQUEEZE

Stretching every 20-30 minutes combats the effects of excessive sitting. It helps avoid the physiological effects of excessive sitting and the associated spinal memory. To perform the appropriate stretch, stand up and reach toward the ceiling (FIGURE 10). Inhale through your nose and exhale through your mouth. During exhalation, stretch higher toward the ceiling. Next, with your palms pointed up, bring your arms down to the side of your body. Then, pretend you are holding a pencil between your shoulder blades and squeeze them together to prevent the pencil from falling. Inhale through your nose and exhale through your mouth. During this exhalation, hold the contraction of your shoulder blades together for 10 seconds (FIGURE 10A). Relax (11, 12). You have successfully completed the basic stretch needed to combat the effects of prolonged sitting. The entire stretch break will not take more than 30 seconds, yet its benefit will last exponentially longer. Repeat this stretch every 20-30 minutes, or as needed.

RELATED NUMBERS: 6-9, 11, 32

11. STAND UP CORRECTLY FROM SITTING

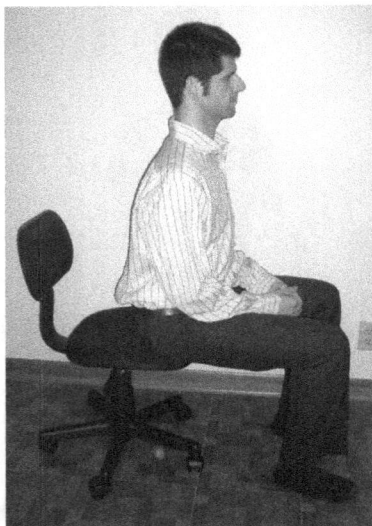

FIG.11

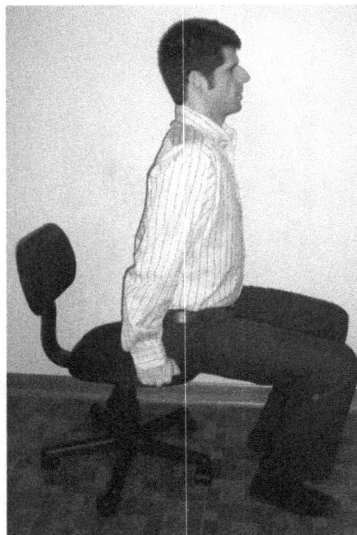

FIG. 11A – MOVE TO EDGE

Standing up correctly from the seated position is one of the most important things I tell patients they can do to spare their backs. It is also one of the easiest. Most people use their low backs to assist them in getting up from the seated position. This is wrong! Think about how many times you get up from sitting. Every time you use your low back to stand, you are flexing your spine and placing unnecessary stress onto it. Here is the easy solution: before you get up from sitting, scoot all the way to the edge of your seated surface, keep your back straight, and get up using your legs, as in FIGURE 11A (12). This may feel strange at first, but should become second nature after a few days. One tip to get started: use your arms to assist your legs in the process (FIGURE 11A). Place your hands into fists and use them to push up off the seated surface, while using your legs. Do not place your fists on your legs. Again, at no time will you flex the low back or use it to assist you in the standing process.

Be sure to not bend your spine—keeping it neutral, as you sit down, too. Simply reverse this standing process, and use the same technique to sit down properly.

RELATED NUMBERS: 6-10, 19, 31-32

12. STAND PROPERLY

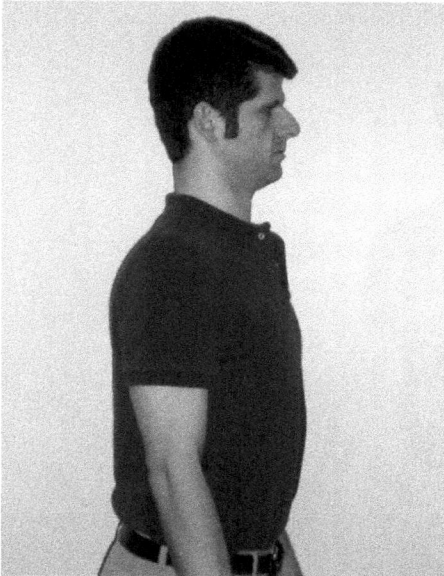

FIG.12 – GOOD POSTURE   FIG.12A – BAD POSTURE

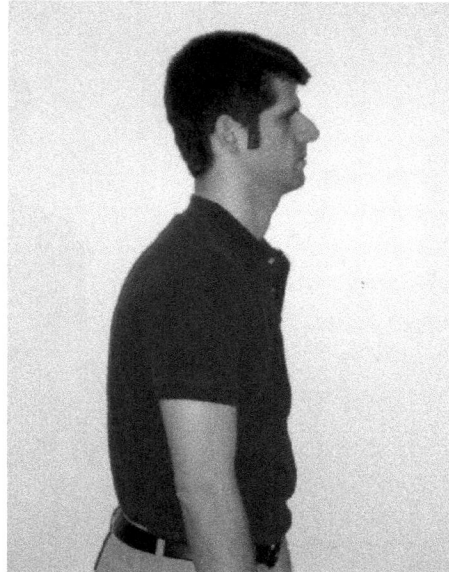

Standing correctly is a foreign concept to most people. This is unfortunate because standing with proper posture is critical to protecting your back and preventing pain and injury. Unlike sitting, I do not believe standing is an inherently damaging position, unless you perform it incorrectly. If you recall, the best seated position is one that changes. I do not recommend sitting in any one position because it is the act of sitting that is harmful (12). Conversely, the act of standing is not harmful if it is done correctly and in moderation.

In order to stand properly, several things must occur. Be sure to ever-so-slightly tuck your head (as discussed with the seated position) so it is in the neutral position. The head is not jutted forward, backward, bent down, or extended backward. The shoulders are retracted backward. An easy way to retract your shoulders is to stand with your arms down to the side with your palms facing backward. From this position, rotate your hands so that your palms are completely facing forward with your thumbs pointing out as far as possible, as in FIGURE 12B.

This end position retracts your shoulders, which is how they should feel in the correct standing posture (12).

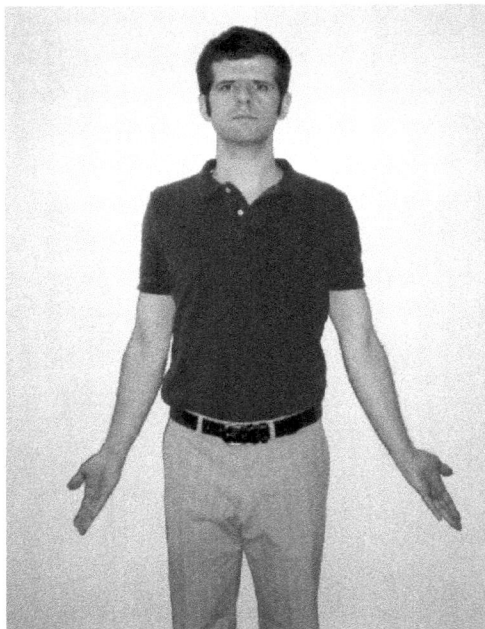

FIG.12B – HOW TO RETRACT YOUR SHOULDERS

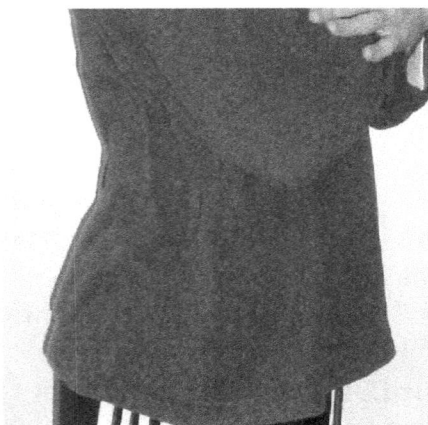

FIG.12C – CORRECT

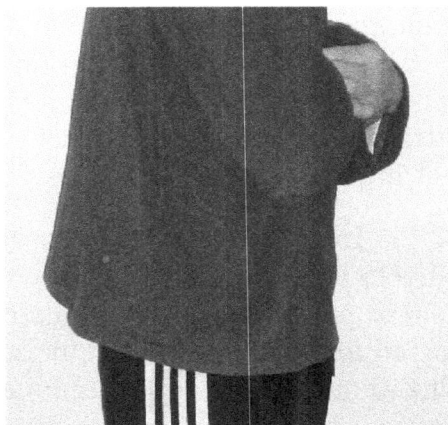

FIG.12D – INCORRECT

Rotate your hips backward. The best way to know if your hips are rotated backward is to look at and feel your low back. With proper hip rotation, the low back will not be flexed, but rather you should see and feel a "ski-slope," or an inverted "C-shape" appearance in the low back (8, 14), as in FIGURE 12C. You should not see and feel a hump, or a "C-shape," in your low back (FIGURE 12D). FIGURE 12D demonstrates improper hip rotation.

RELATED NUMBERS: 13-14, 32

13. DON'T STAND TOO LONG

As mentioned, I don't believe excessive standing is as much of a problem as excessive sitting. However, standing can lead to chronic low back pain. To combat the potential effects of standing too long, I recommend taking a break from standing after every 20-30 minutes. Excessive standing is typically considered 50 minutes or longer, but I recommend 20-30 minutes because of spinal memory (secret #4) (12). If your job or lifestyle requires prolonged standing, bring a stool to your workstation. I suggest sitting for a minute or two every 20-30 minutes. Combining a rest break after 50 minutes, and sitting every 20-30 minutes is a great way to avoid the effects of excessive standing.

Another suggestion is to switch your weight-bearing foot. Every 10-15 minutes, switch your weight to your right foot. Stand with your weight on the right foot for one minute. Then, switch the weight to your left foot for one minute. Next, stand normally with the weight equally distributed on both feet. In another 10-15 minutes, switch weight-bearing feet again and repeat the process. A different way to accomplish this same concept is with a small step stool. Place the non weight-bearing foot on the small step stool and alternate feet as previously described (8). There is no set rule to how frequently you should switch weight-bearing feet. Do what makes you feel best.

RELATED NUMBERS: 12, 14, 32

14. ROCK BACKWARD AND FORWARD WHILE STANDING

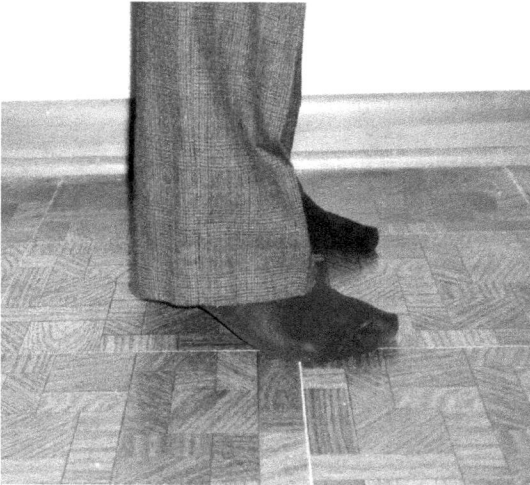

FIG.14 – FORWARD   FIG.14A – BACKWARD

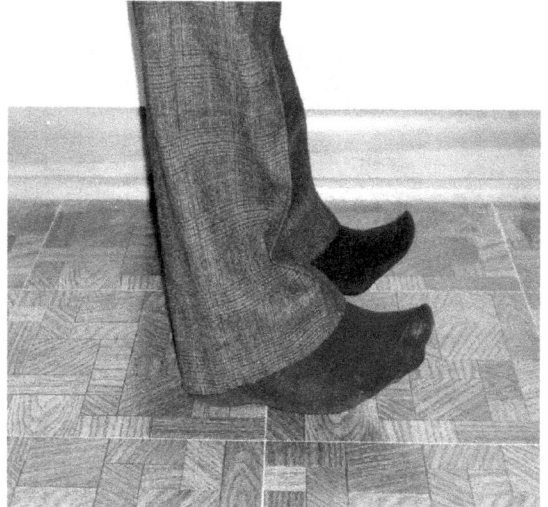

Evidence shows that you can develop chronic low back pain from excessive standing. This chronic low back pain seems to result from a lack of movement, specifically forward and backward, while standing. As a result, I suggest rocking backward and forward on the balls and heels of your feet (10). Please refer to FIGURES 14 and 14A. Rocking backward and forward is not something you do constantly. I recommend every five minutes you rock backward and forward for about 60 seconds. Again, there is no rule set in stone as to the frequency with which you should rock forward and backward, as it is based on your feeling.

RELATED NUMBERS: 12-13

15. POSITION YOUR COMPUTER MONITOR CORRECTLY

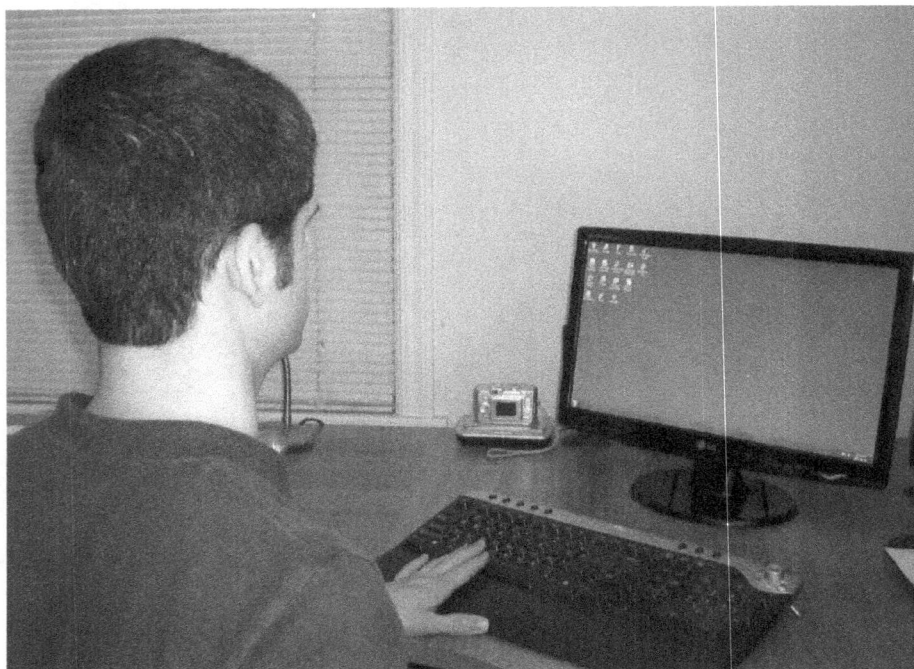

FIGURE 15 – CORRECT POSITIONING

Hopefully, you don't sit at a computer for longer than 50 minutes. However, if you do, make sure the computer monitor is positioned appropriately to prevent any back problems. Be certain the monitor is positioned so that there is no glare on the screen. Second, place the monitor so that your head is not too far forward or backward, and you don't have to squint while looking at the screen (8, 11, 14).

RELATED NUMBERS: 6, 16, 32

16. DO NOT SIT WITH SHRUGGED SHOULDERS

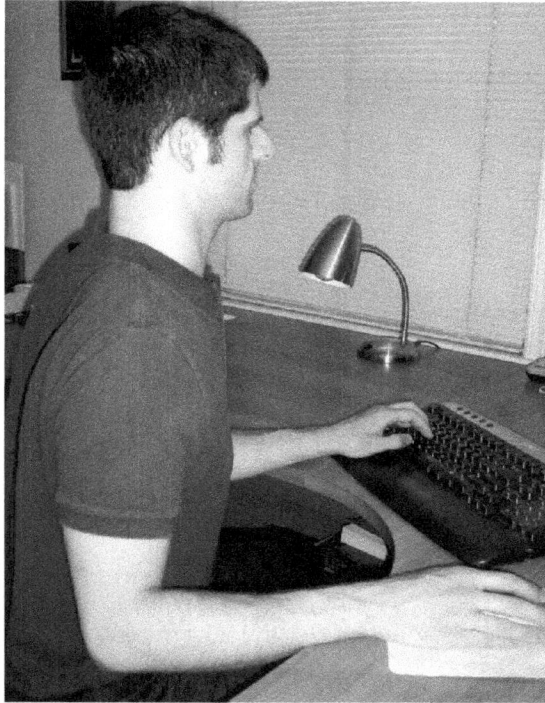

FIGURE 16 – CORRECT POSITIONING

Make sure your work station does not force you to sit with shrugged shoulders (FIGURE 16). If you use a keyboard, it should not be elevated so that your shoulders are in a perpetually shrugged position. Likewise, do not use an elevated desk or rest your elbows on the desk or arms of the chair, as this forces shrugged shoulders. The desk height cannot typically be altered, which is why it is important to use an ergonomic chair that can be raised and lowered accordingly (8, 11).

RELATED NUMBERS: 6-9, 15, 32

17. USE A BOOK STAND WHEN READING

 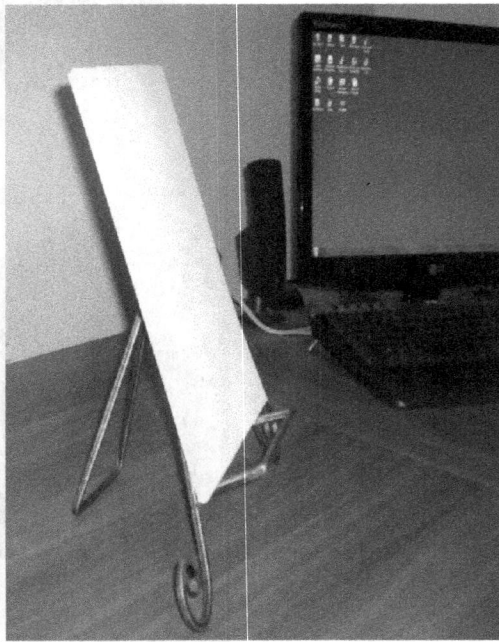

FIGURE 17   FIGURE 17A

When you read, do not bend your head too far forward and down. To prevent improperly positioning your head while you read, use a book stand or an inclined reading surface. An incline of 12 degrees is enough to prevent the ill-effects of a bent head posture. However, many tables and reading surfaces are not made with this incline, so it is easier to purchase a book stand to hold your reading material upright (FIGURE 17 and 17A). A bookstand reduces possible muscle spasms, headaches, and pain from prolonged improper head positioning (8, 14).

You can find links for book stands to purchase at **www.backsafetyandwellness.com/products**.

RELATED NUMBERS: 6, 32

18. USE A PHONE HEADSET

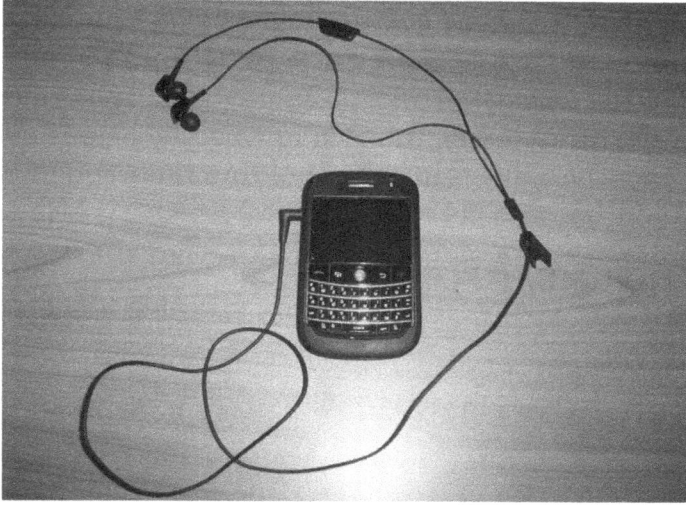

FIGURE 18 – CORRECT

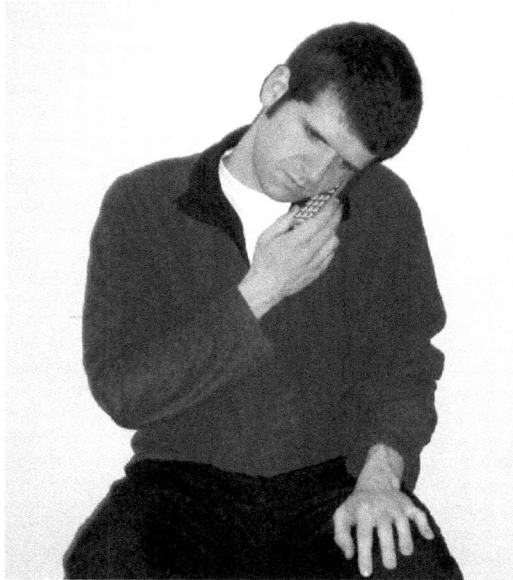

FIGURE 18A – INCORRECT

Using a phone headset eliminates the possibility of torticollis, or muscles spasms in the neck, from improper phone usage. Repeatedly bending your head to your shoulder to hold a phone causes injury to the joints, muscles, and ligaments in the neck (FIGURE 18A). It is also possible for injuries to these areas to cause referral pain and subsequent headaches. If use of a headset is not possible, alternate holding the phone with your right and left hand (8, 11, 12).

RELATED NUMBERS: 32

19. SIT PROPERLY IN THE CAR

Back injury is common from sitting incorrectly in the car. The driver's and passenger's seats must allow for the most ideal seated position. I do not recommend the driver or passenger try to maintain a dynamic seated position while driving. It is safer for the driver and passenger to ensure their seat is set for the most ideal seated position possible. The driver's and passenger's seats should allow for the legs and hips to be at 90 degrees. Use a lumbar support (**www.backsafetyandwellness.com/products**) to avoid forming the "C shape," or hump, in the low back. Instead, a ski slope, or inverted "C-shape," is desired. Please refer to FIGURE 6. Do not flex the low back!

Do not shrug your shoulders. Some people place their arms on the door rest, which causes a constant shoulder shrug. Avoid this. In addition, drivers tend to place one arm on the steering wheel and shift their weight to one side. Again, try to avoid this. Rather, place both hands on the steering wheel. The arms and elbows, if possible, should be at 90 degrees.

FIGURE 19 – PROPER HEAD POSITION

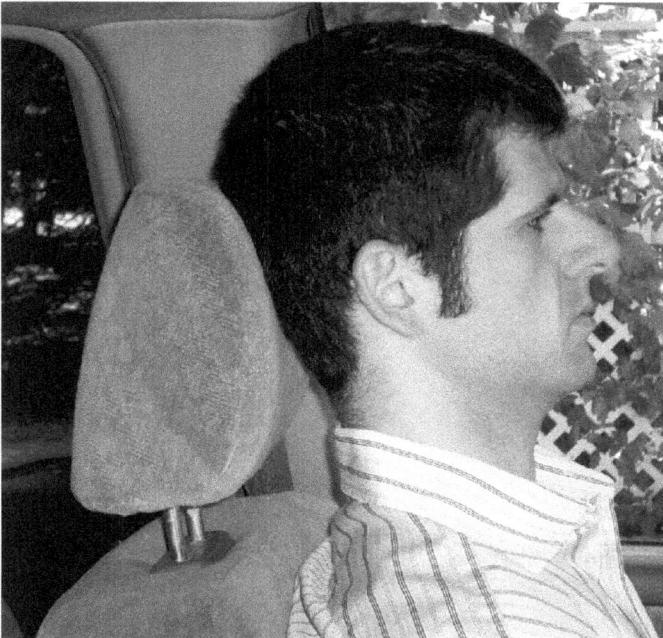

Do not position the head rest too far forward. Ideally, your head should rest against the head rest at the spot directly above the bump on the back of the head. If properly positioned, your head will appear slightly bent backward at 15-20 degrees as in FIGURE 19 (11, 14).

The passenger should follow the same guidelines as the driver. Properly sitting in the car will allow you and your passenger to feel better after a long drive.

RELATED NUMBERS: 6-7, 11, 20

20. GET IN AND OUT OF THE CAR CORRECTLY

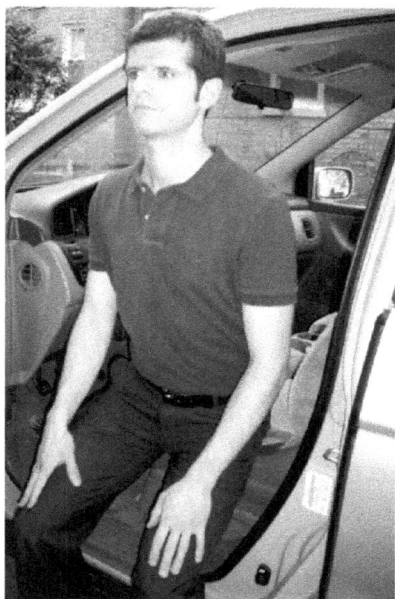

FIGURE 20 – STEP ONE

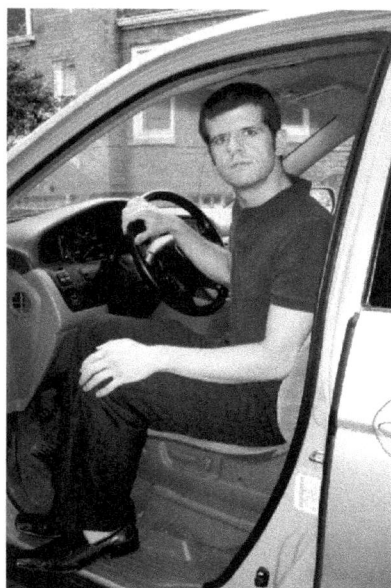

FIGURE 20A – STEP TWO

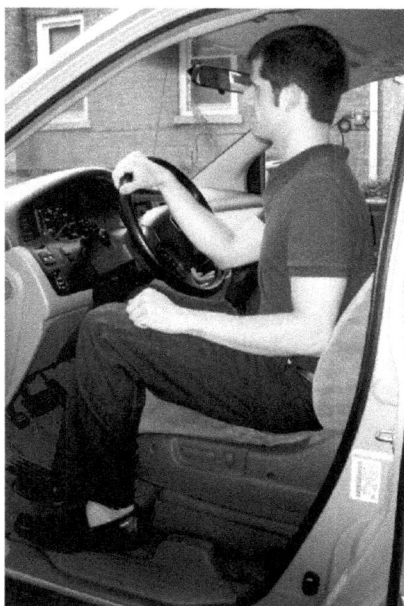

FIGURE 20B – EXITING

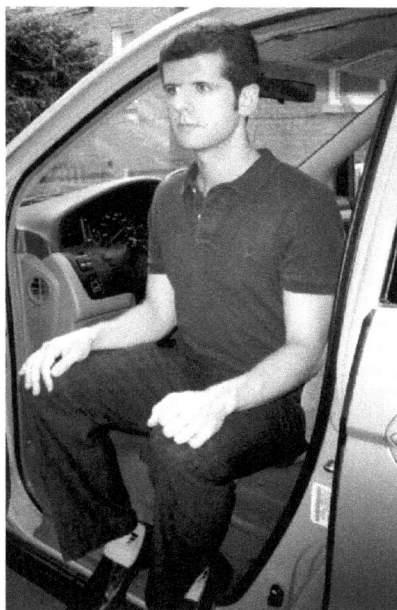

FIGURE 20C – EXITING

Getting into and out of the car incorrectly can easily harm your back. Unfortunately, some people have jobs and lifestyles that require frequent trips into and out of their automobiles. These people are likely hurting their backs and don't know it. The correct way to get into your car is to stand with your buttocks towards the car door. From this position, squat or use hip rotation (secret #'s 33 and 34) to step backwards into the car seat (FIGURE 20). Then, swing your legs around to the front of the car (FIGURE 20A). The incorrect way to get into the car is to stand sideways next to the door, bend away from the car, and plop into the seat.

You will get out of the car the same way as you entered it, but in the opposite order that you entered it. First, swing your legs around from the front of the car to the side (FIGURE 20B). Next, scoot all the way towards the edge of the seat and get up using your legs, not your back (FIGURE 20C). This method spares your back and decreases the risk of injury (11, 12).

RELATED NUMBERS: 6, 11, 19

21. WALK QUICKLY

Walking is an essential part of life. Let's make sure you do it in the most efficient manner and protect your back. Walking quickly, as opposed to a slower walking pace, leads to a shorter recovery time for low back disorders and aids in prevention of future back problems. Conversely, walking slowly may actually cause low back problems and worsen the symptoms of a current problem (11, 12, 14).

RELATED NUMBERS: 12, 22

22. SWING YOUR ARMS WHILE YOU WALK

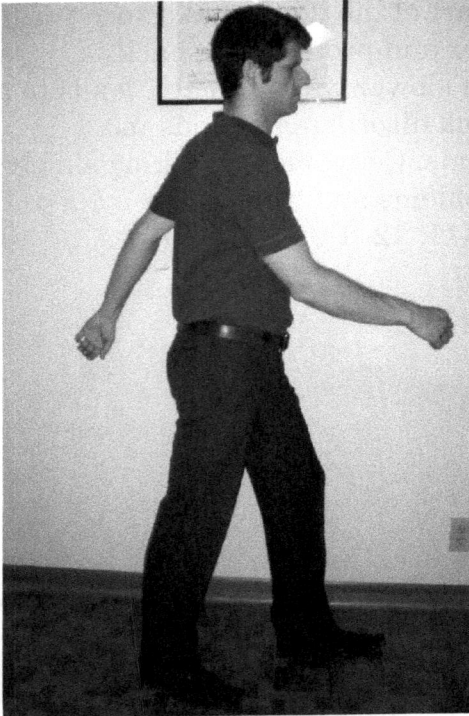

FIGURE 22 – GOOD   FIGURE 22A – BAD

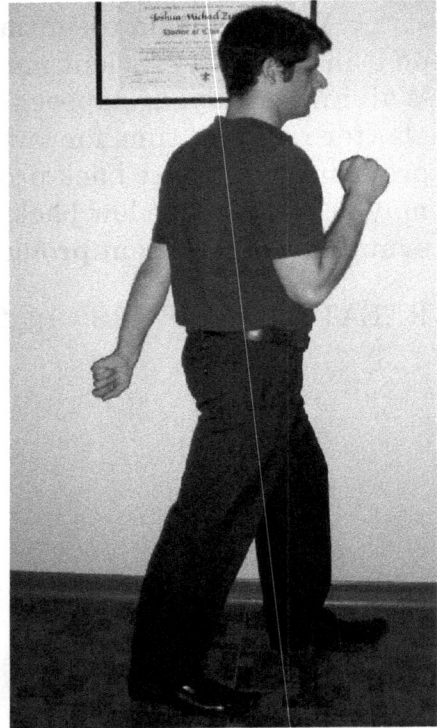

Some people do not move their arms while they walk. Sadly, these people not only look odd while they walk, but they are hurting their low backs, too. Swinging your arms while you walk decreases stresses on the spine by 10%. Be certain you are swinging your arms from your shoulders (FIGURE 22), and not your elbows (FIGURE 22A). Arm swinging from the elbows does not demonstrate the same benefit as arm swinging from the shoulders (12).

RELATED NUMBERS: 12, 21

23. BREATHE PROPERLY

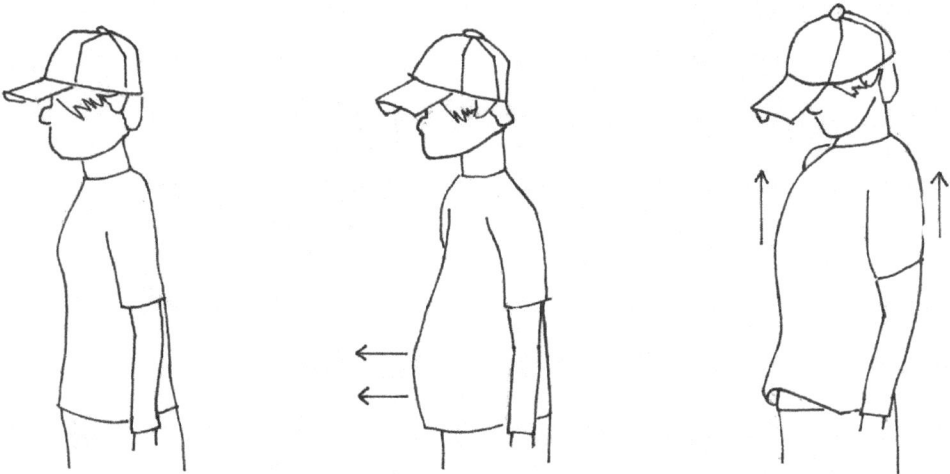

FIG.23*   FIG.23A – GOOD*   FIG.23B – BAD*

Believe it or not, there is a right and wrong way to breathe. The proper way to breathe in air, or inhale, involves using a muscle called the diaphragm. When you properly inhale, you should naturally stick out your stomach and widen your ribcage (FIGURE 23A). However, some people will inhale incorrectly by raising their shoulders, or shrugging them, instead of sticking out their stomach (FIGURE 23B). The latter example does not use the diaphragm and should be avoided. Each time you inhale, push out your stomach using your diaphragm to widen the ribcage. Avoid use of the shoulders or chest, as in FIGURE 23B.

The proper way to exhale, or breathe out air, is to suck the stomach in towards the spine. People typically do not exhale incorrectly. An example of improper exhalation is sticking out the stomach as you breathe out the air. Sticking out the stomach as you exhale throws off the biomechanics of the body. Breathing incorrectly can cause low back and neck pain (11).

*illustrations courtesy of Eric Dangoy

24. DON'T SIT ON YOUR WALLET

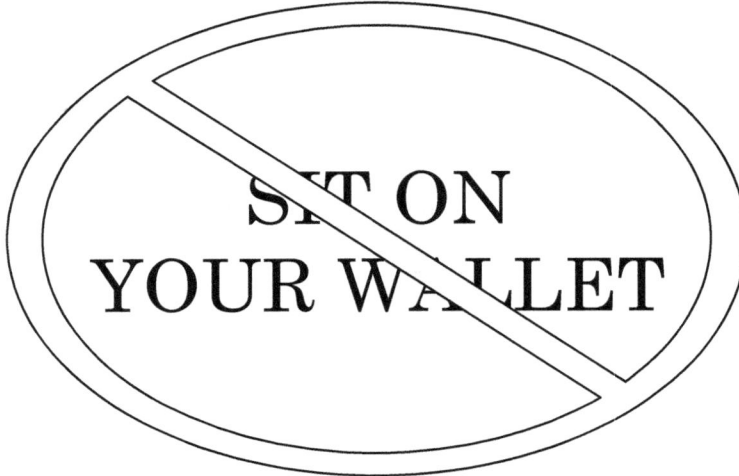

SIT ON YOUR WALLET

Most men keep their wallet in their back pocket and, as a result, sit on their wallets. I don't recommend sitting on your wallet. I believe it throws off the pelvis, makes the pelvis unlevel, and alters the spine. No one wants to sit on an unlevel chair, yet that is essentially what happens each time you sit on your wallet. Place your wallet in your front pocket, or remove it from your pants when you sit. Be balanced when you sit.

I recommend using a slim, "back-sparing" wallet that fits comfortably in your front pocket. You can find a "back-sparing" wallet at **www.backsafetyandwellness.com/products**.

RELATED NUMBERS: 6-11, 32

25. AVOID WEARING HIGH HEELS

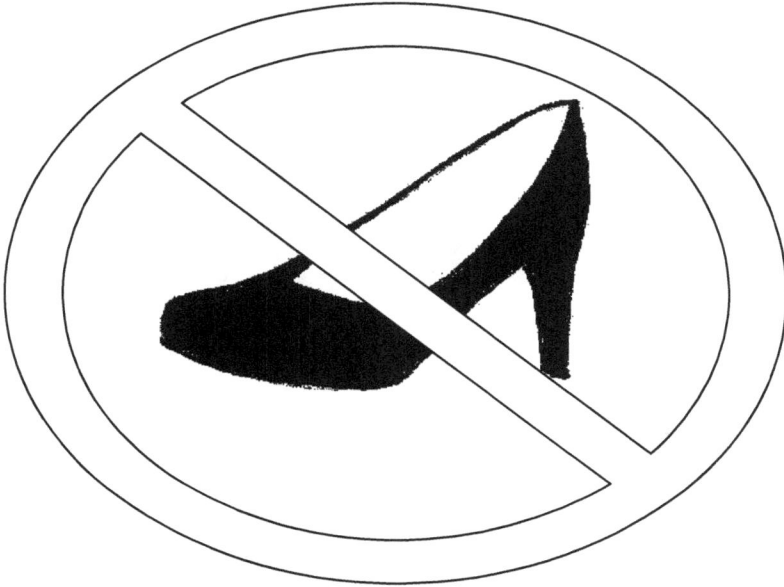

I'm not making a lot of women happy with this recommendation, but it's the truth: avoid high heels. High heels increase the stresses placed on your low back joints, may alter your gait, and disrupt the overall biomechanics of your body. High heels also cause bunions and hammer toes (14). If avoiding high heels is too difficult, at least minimize your use of them. Flat, cushioned shoes are better for your back. Reduce your use of high heels to prevent a sore back and imperfect feet!

RELATED NUMBERS: 32

26. AVOID VIBRATION

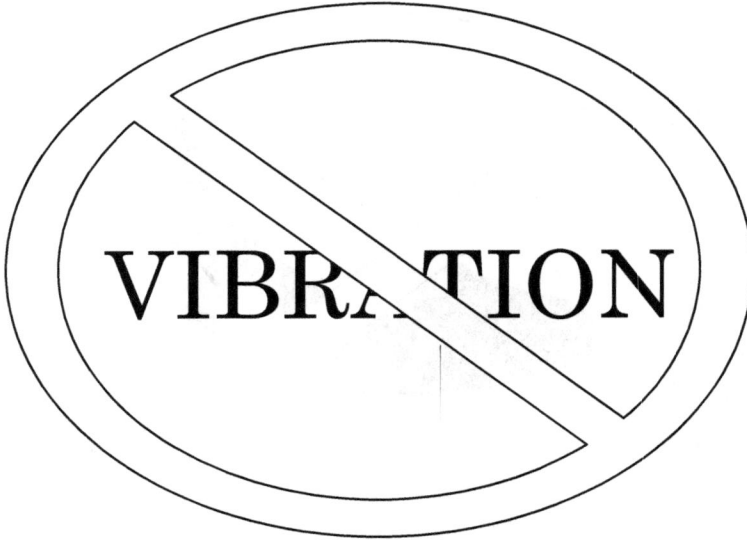

VIBRATION

Seated, whole-body vibration is linked to a higher likelihood of low back disorders. Some professions require sustained whole-body vibration, so in these instances be sure to change positions, take frequent breaks, and use a lumbar support. The effects of whole-body vibration are minimized if you sit with proper posture, while exposed to the vibration, and decrease the exposure time of the whole-body vibration (15, 17). See "secret" #6 for the "ideal seated position" and "secret" #7 for lumbar supports.

RELATED NUMBERS: 6-7, 32

27. USE A MEDIUM-FIRM MATTRESS

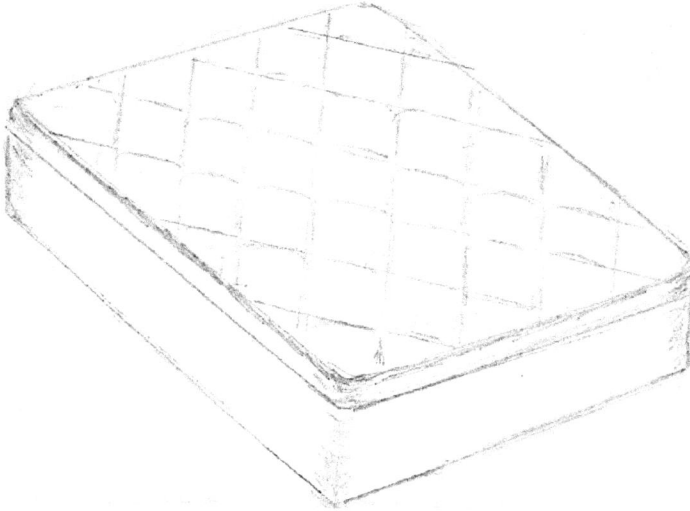

Studies reveal the mattress you sleep on affects your comfort. There is a correlation between sleeping surfaces, sleep discomfort, and associated pain. A medium-firm mattress is the most desirable. Your mattress should not be too firm or too soft. The average person can decrease sleep discomfort and enjoy a better, pain-free night's rest simply by changing his or her mattress (4, 5, 7).

In addition, make sure your mattress is not too old. Mattresses that are around 10 years old may result in discomfort and pain after sleep. Additional research shows that discomfort is significantly reduced when a new mattress is used (6). I know it's expensive to purchase a new mattress every 10 years, but it seems to make a difference. If purchasing a mattress every 10 years is not possible, at least flip and rotate your mattress yearly.

RELATED NUMBERS: 28-31

28. USE A CERVICAL PILLOW

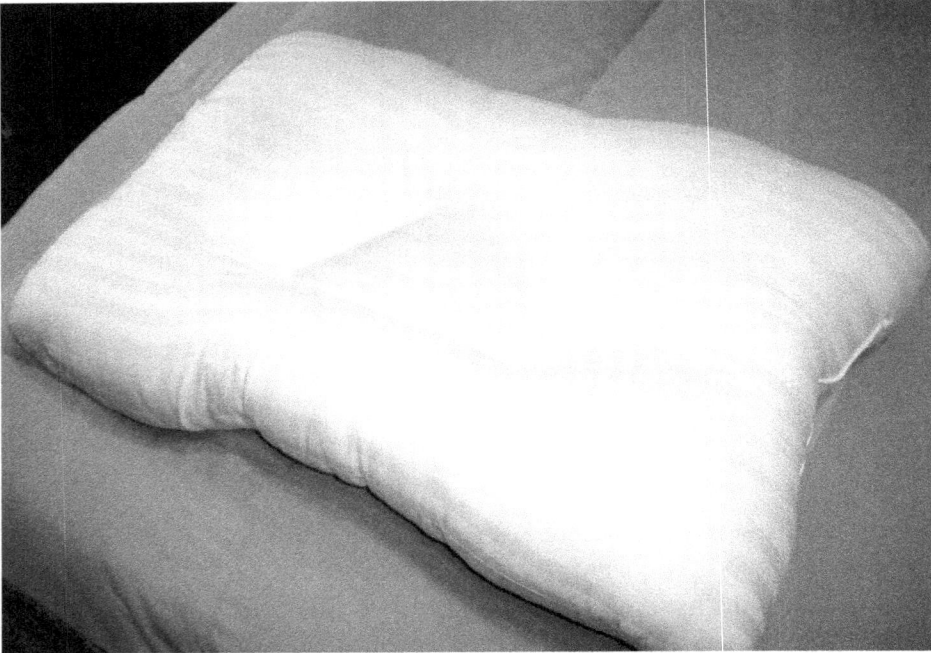

FIGURE 28 – CERVICAL PILLOW

Most pillows do not support the shape of the neck. As a result, your neck becomes irritated from the lack of support (8). A cervical pillow, pictured in FIGURE 28, is designed to support your neck, prevent soreness upon awaking, and maintain the neck's shape. The ideal pillow is not too hard, not too high, hypoallergenic, washable, and maintains the neck's curve. Most feather pillows do not allow for proper neck support (1, 16). Use a cervical pillow to avoid any possible neck pain upon waking, and subsequent headaches.

Visit **www.backsafetyandwellness.com/products** to find my recommended cervical pillows.

RELATED NUMBERS: 27, 29-31

29. NO STOMACH SLEEPING

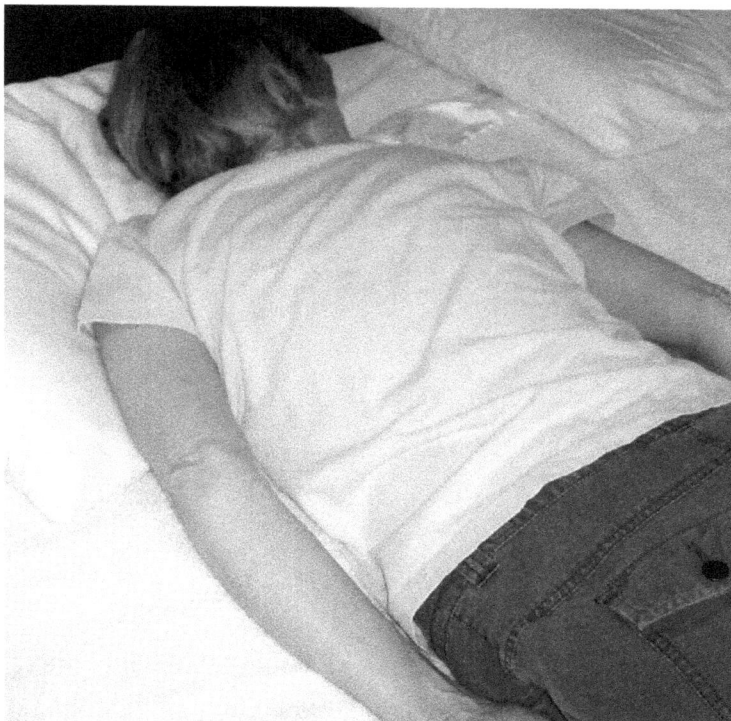

FIGURE 29 – AVOID STOMACH SLEEPING

You should not sleep on your stomach (11, 14). Stomach sleeping is one potential cause of waking up with neck pain, low back pain, and headaches as it does not allow the spine to maintain its ideal, natural curves. See "secret" #30 for alternatives.

RELATED NUMBERS: 27-28, 30-31

30. SLEEP ON YOUR SIDE OR BACK

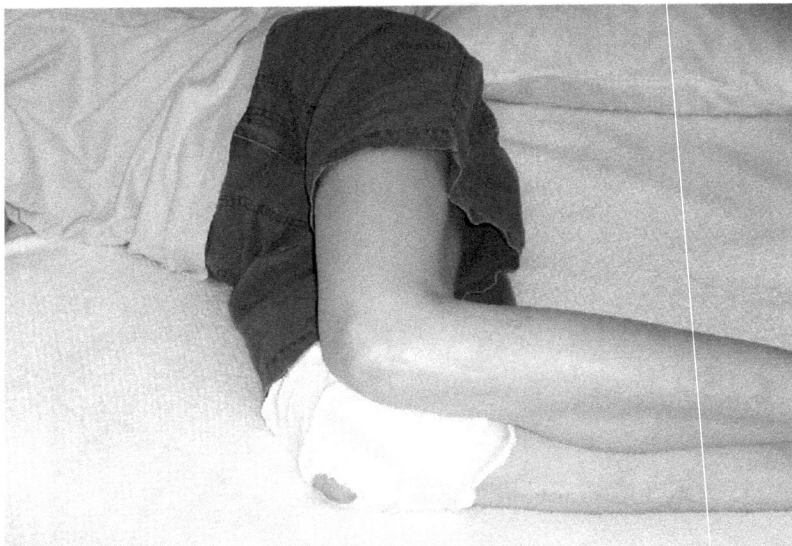

FIGURE 30 – GOOD

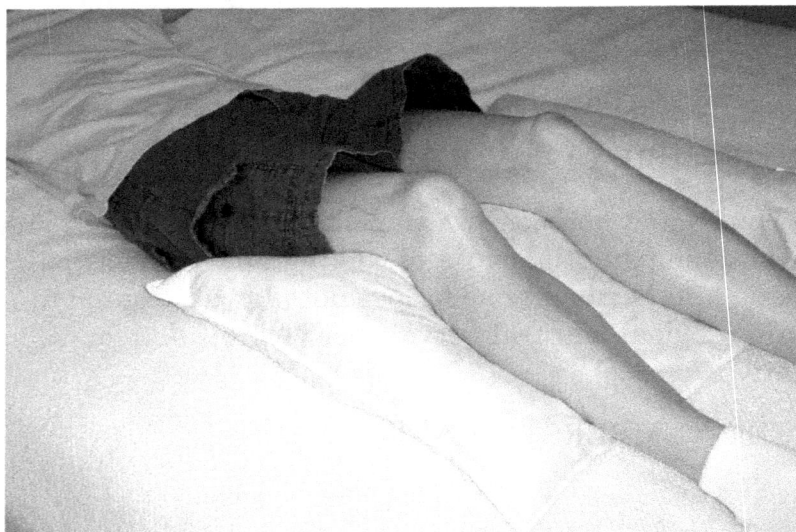

FIGURE 30A – GOOD

Sleeping on your side and back are both perfectly acceptable (3). However, if you sleep on your side, place a pillow between your knees, as in FIGURE 30 (8, 11, 14). When you sleep on your side, the knees have a tendency to rest atop one another and create discomfort while you sleep. Placing a pillow between your knees should eliminate the knee discomfort and ensure the spine's natural curves are intact. You can find side-sleeping pillows on my website at **www.backsafetyandwellness.com/products**.

Similarly, if you choose to sleep on your back, I recommend placing a pillow underneath your knees, as in FIGURE 30A (8, 11, 14). Back and side sleeping may reduce the natural curves in your spine and cause discomfort overnight (14). These recommendations can prevent low back pain. Although sleeping on your side and back are not inherently perfect, there are ways to make it ideal.

RELATED NUMBERS: 27-29, 31

31. GET OUT OF BED CORRECTLY

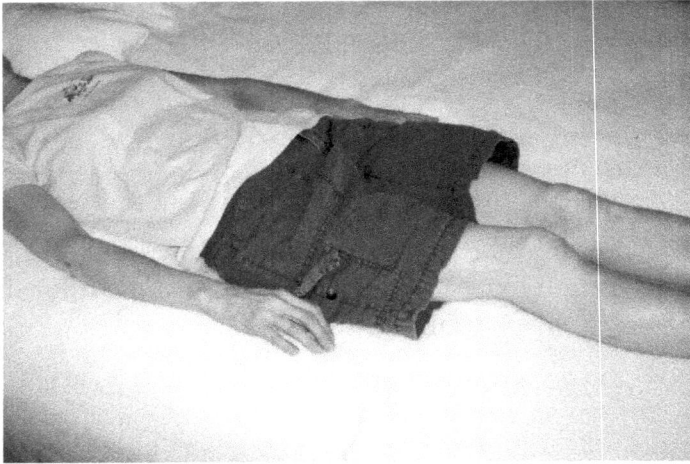

FIGURE 31 – STEP 1

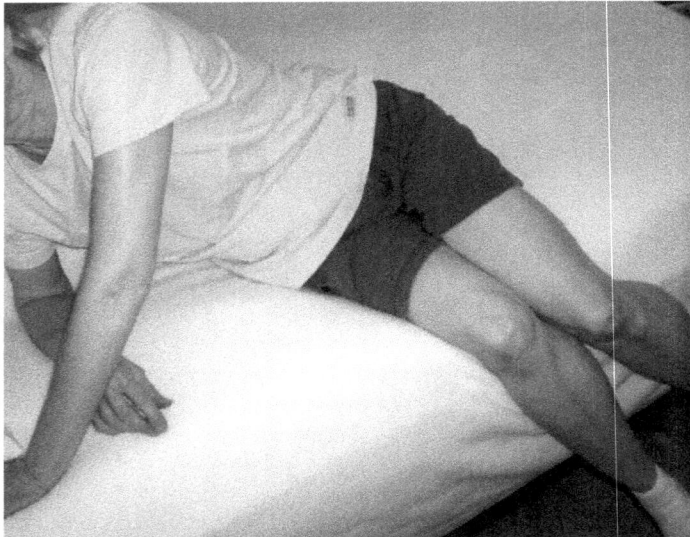

FIGURE 31A – STEP 2

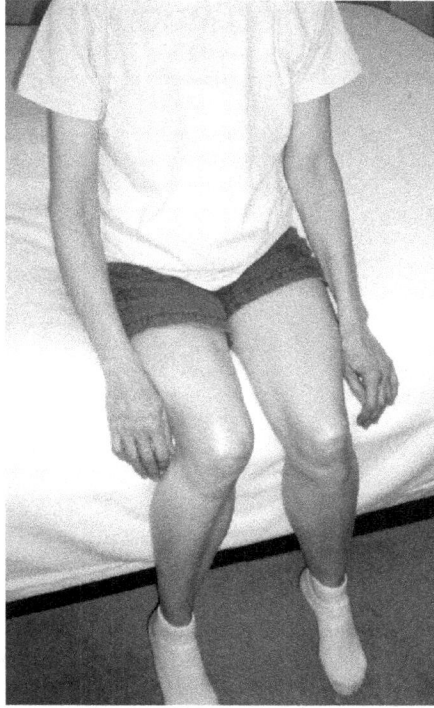

FIGURE 31B – STEP 3

  Your bed should be a relaxing place, where you go to prepare for a new day and forget your troubles. Your bed should not be a source of pain. Unfortunately, patients tell me far too often that they dread going to bed because it hurts too much to get out of it. Whether you have back pain or not, make sure you are getting out of bed correctly. Most people sit up and then twist their backs to get out bed, which is wrong. To get out of bed correctly, I recommend rolling onto your side, while you are still lying down, and sitting up from the side lying position (FIGURE 31A). From there, scoot to the edge of the bed, stand up without bending your back, and use your legs to stand (FIGURE 31B). This method spares your back (11).

RELATED NUMBERS: 1, 3, 11, 27-30

32. DON'T DO TOO MUCH OF ANY ONE THING

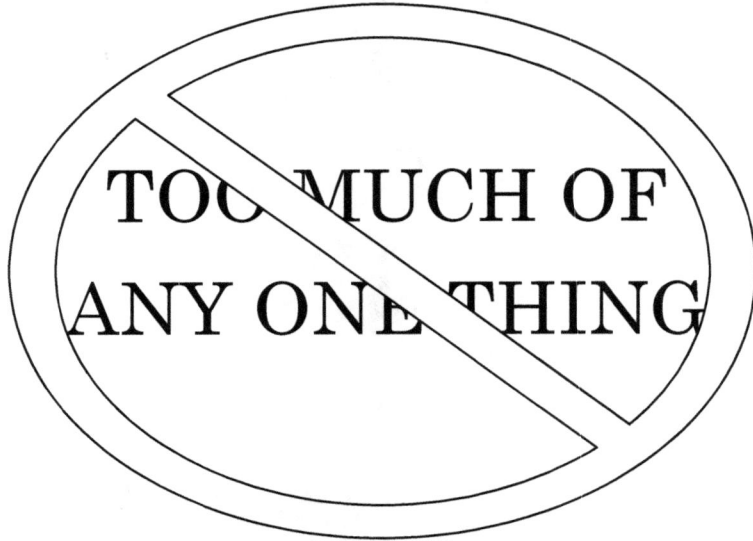

TOO MUCH OF ANY ONE THING

Whether it is sitting, standing, twisting, or bending, the premise is the same. Don't do too much of any one thing. Performing the same movement repeatedly harms the body. The body likes symmetry and change. If some of my recommendations are not feasible for your job or lifestyle, do your best to change the order of your tasks (12). For example, switch the placement of your phone from the left side of your desk to the right side every other week, if you are unable to use a headset. Change your sitting position. Take rest breaks. It is little things like these that protect the body from overuse and injury. Recall that excessive sitting or standing occurs after 50 minutes, so remember to take your stretch breaks.

REFERENCES

1. Gordon, S.J., et al. "Pillow Use: The Behaviour of Cervical Pain, Sleep Quality, and Pillow Comfort in Side Sleepers." Manual Therapy 14.6 (2009): 671-78. Print.

2. Gregory, D.E., et al. "Stability Ball Versus Office Chair: Comparison of Muscle Activation and Lumbar Spine Posture During Prolonged Sitting." Human Factors 48.1 (2006): 142-53. Print.

3. Huff, Lew, and David M. Brady. *Instant Access to Chiropractic Guidelines and Protocols.* 2nd ed. St. Louis: Elsevier Mosby, 2005. Print.

4. Jacobson, B.H., et al. "Changes in Back Pain, Sleep Quality, and Perceived Stress After Introduction of New Bedding Systems." Journal of Chiropractic Medicine 8.1 (2009): 1-8. Print.

5. Jacobson, B.H., et al. "Effect of Prescribed Sleep Surfaces on Back Pain and Sleep Quality in Patients Diagnosed with Low Back and Shoulder Pain." Applied Ergonomics 42.1 (2010): 91-97. Print.

6. Jacobson, B.H., et al. "Grouped Comparisons of Sleep Quality for New and Personal Bedding Systems." Applied Ergonomics 39.2 (2008): 247-54. Print.

7. Jacobson, B.H., et al. "Subjective Rating of Perceived Back Pain, Stiffness, and Sleep Quality Following Introduction of Medium-Firm Bedding Systems." Journal of Chiropractic Medicin. 5.4 (2006): 128-34. Print.

8. Khalil, Tarek M., et al. *Ergonomics in Back Pain: A Guide to Prevention and Rehabilitation.* New York: Van Nostrand Reinhold, 1993. Print.

9. Kingma, I., et al. "Static and Dynamic Postural Loadings During Computer Work in Females: Sitting on an Office Chair Versus Sitting on an Exericse Ball." Applied Ergonomics 40.2 (2009): 199-205. Print.

10. Lafond, D., et al. "Postural Control during Prolonged Standing in Persons with Chronic Low Back Pain." Gait Posture 29.3 (2009): 421-27. Print.

11. Liebenson, Craig. *Rehabilitation of the Spine: A Practitioners Manual.* 2nd ed. Baltimore: Lippincott, 2007. Print.

12. McGill, Stuart. *Low Back Disorders: Evidence-based Prevention and Rehabilitation.* 2nd ed. Champaign: Human Kinetics, 2007. Print.

13. McGill, Stuart, et al. "Sitting on a Chair or an Exercise Ball: Various Perspectives to Guide Decision Making." Clinical Biomechanics 21.4 (2006): 353-60. Print.

14. Nordin, Margareta, and Victor H. Frankel. *Basic Biomechanics of the Musculoskeletal System.* 3rd ed. Baltimore: Lippincott, 2001. Print.

15. Okunribido, O.O., et al. "The Role of Whole Body Vibration, Posture and Manual Materials Handling as Risk Factors for Low Back Pain in Occupational Drivers." Ergonomics 51.3 (2008): 308-29. Print.

16. Persson, L., and U. Moritz. "Neck Support Pillows: A Comparative Study." Journal of Manipulative and Physiological Therapeutics 21.4 (1998): 237-40. Print.
17. Pope, M.H., et al. "A Review of Studies on Seated Whole Body Vibration and Low Back Pain." Proceedings of the Institution of Mechanical Engineers. Part H, Journal of Engineering in Medicine 213.6 (1999): 435-46. Print.

CHAPTER 2: TASKS

33. USE HIP ROTATION

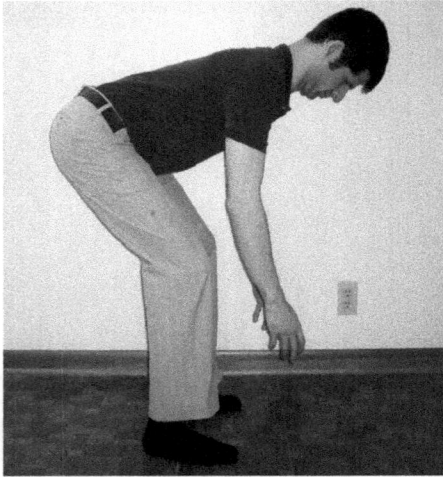

FIG.33 – GOOD

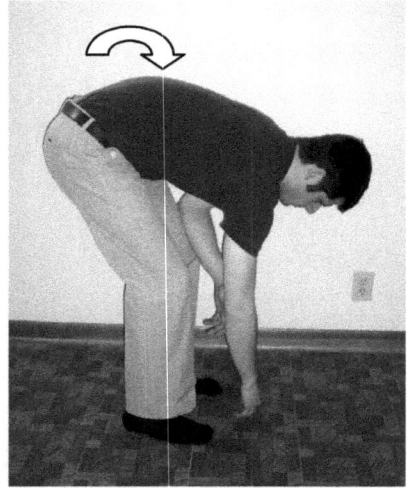

FIG.33A – AVOID THIS

A key concept in protecting your spine is to NOT bend with your back, but to rotate with your hips. Hip rotation is an alternative to flexing your spine to bend or to pick up an object. It is frequently combined with a squat, when you have to pick up a large object. Most people, when they bend down, use their back, as in FIGURE 33A. This is incorrect. Notice our enemy, the "C-shaped" hump in the low back, in FIGURE 33A. The proper way to bend or pick up something is to rotate about your hips, keeping your back straight, and bending your knees if necessary. Imagine there is a horizontal axis that runs from one hip, through your pelvis, to the opposite hip. Your hips should rotate forward about this imaginary axis, while keeping the back straight, to pick up something from the floor, and each time you bend (FIGURE 33). Using hip rotation spares the spine of harmful work.

The important thing to remember when performing hip rotation is to first stick out your butt. Next, keep your back neutral (straight) and keep the object as close to your body as possible. From there, rotate your hips and spare your back (2, 4).

RELATED NUMBERS: 1, 2, 34-35

34. USE A SQUAT

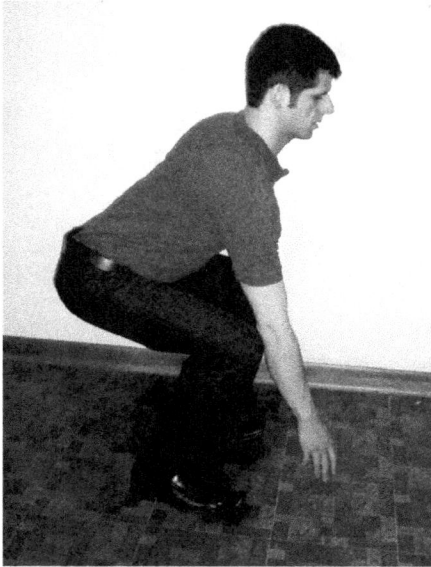

FIG.34 – GOOD, NO C-SHAPE

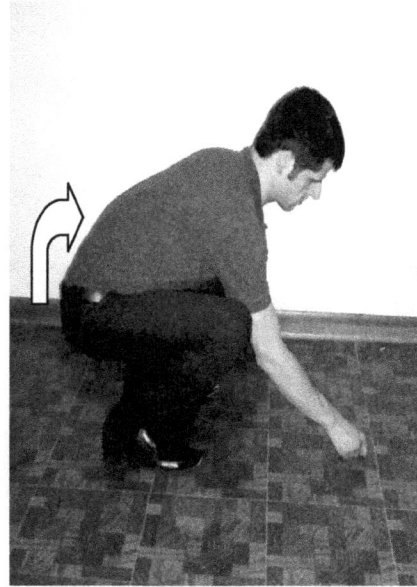

FIG.34A – BAD, C-SHAPE

A second alternative to flexing the spine when you lift an object or bend is a squat. Squats are best for not damaging your back when lifting heavier objects. To properly perform a squat, keep your spine neutral, or straight, do not bend your knees past 90 degrees, and keep the object that you are picking up close to your body (FIGURE 34). When performing a squat, keep in mind the three "N's": ninety—don't bend your knees past 90 degrees, near—keep the object near to your body, and neutral—do not bend your back (2, 4). FIGURE 34A shows the incorrect way to squat. Note the "C-shaped" hump in the back, indicating flexion of the spine.

RELATED NUMBERS: 1-2, 33, 35

35. USE A GOLFER'S LIFT

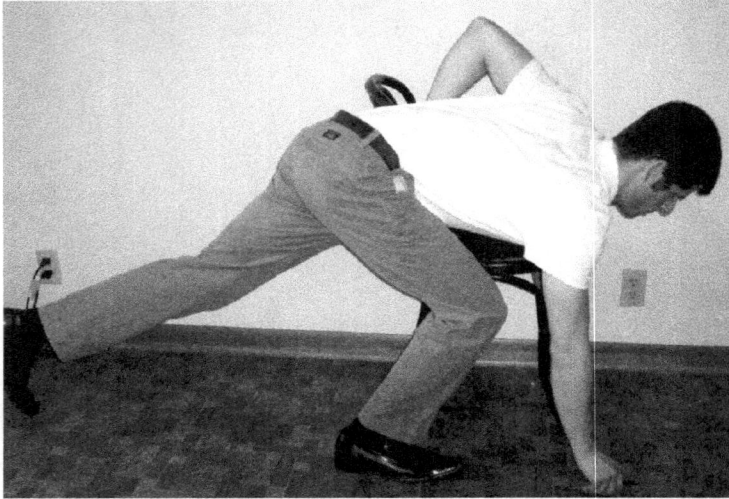

FIGURE 35 – PROPER GOLFER'S LIFT

You want to avoid flexion of your spine at all times. However, most tasks require bending of some kind, which makes it impossible to avoid flexion completely. A third alternative to flexing your spine is a golfer's lift. A golfer's lift is best used for frequent bending and lifting of light items. To properly perform a golfer's lift, rotate your hips, keep your back neutral, bend one of your knees, and use the unbent leg as a counterweight to balance yourself (FIGURE 35). Do not use the same knee to bend every time, and alternate between the left and right leg to balance. You may find it easier to hold on to something for support (4).

RELATED NUMBERS: 1-2, 33-34

36. LIFT OBJECTS CLOSE TO YOUR BODY

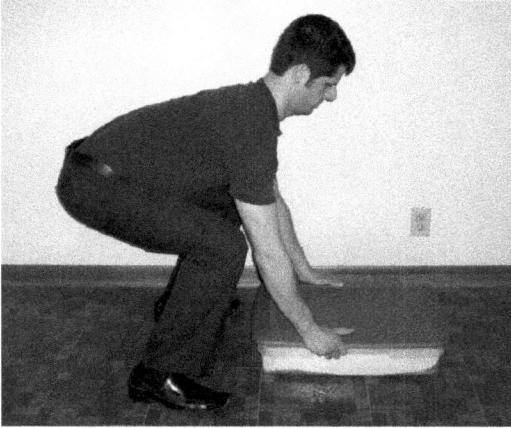

FIGURE 36 – GOOD   FIGURE 36A – BAD

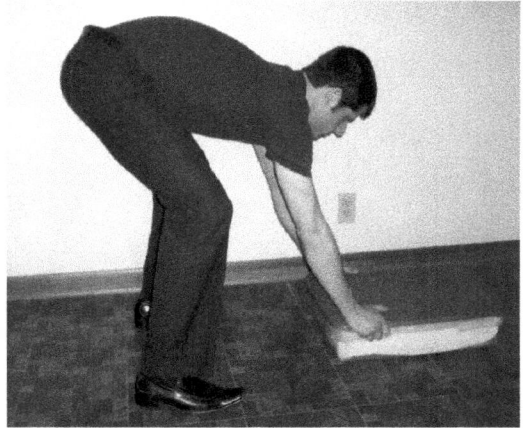

Anytime you lift an object, make sure it is close to your body. Bend forward appropriately using a squat, golfer's lift, hip rotation, or combination of the three to pick up the object. Then, keep it as close to your body as possible as you lift it (FIGURE 36). When you pick up an object from far away, it places stress on the low back, as in FIGURE 36A (1, 2, 4, 6).

RELATED NUMBERS: 1, 33-35, 37

37. PICK UP CHILDREN CORRECTLY

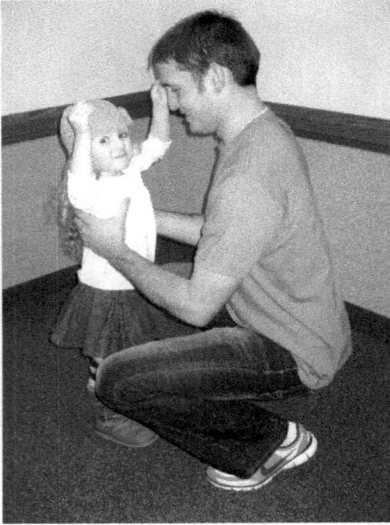
FIG.37 – GOOD

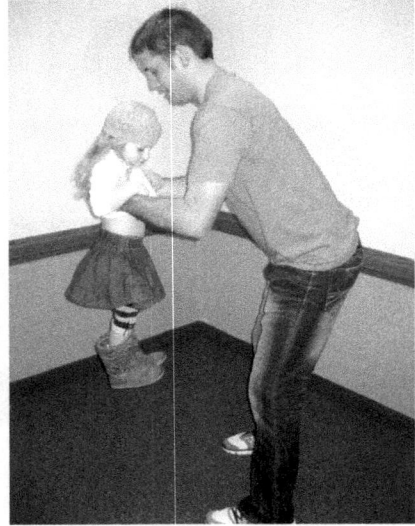
FIG.37A – GOOD

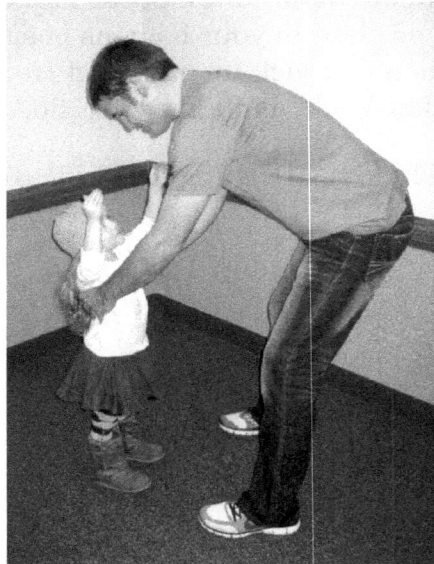
FIGURE 37B – BAD

The majority of my patients admit they've hurt their backs doing one thing: picking up children. Parents, grandparents, and daycare workers will likely agree that picking up children at some point has hurt their backs. Why? People perform it incorrectly! Don't worry, with three simple steps, you'll pick up beckoning children painlessly more times than you'll want. First, get close to the child and squat down correctly, as shown in FIGURE 37. Then, use proper hip rotation to bring the child close to your body and stand (FIGURE 37A). Avoid using your back to pick up the child (FIGURE 37B). If performed correctly, you've kept a neutral (straight) spine and didn't use your back to pick up the child.

RELATED NUMBERS: 1-2, 33-36

38. PICK UP GROCERY BAGS CORRECTLY

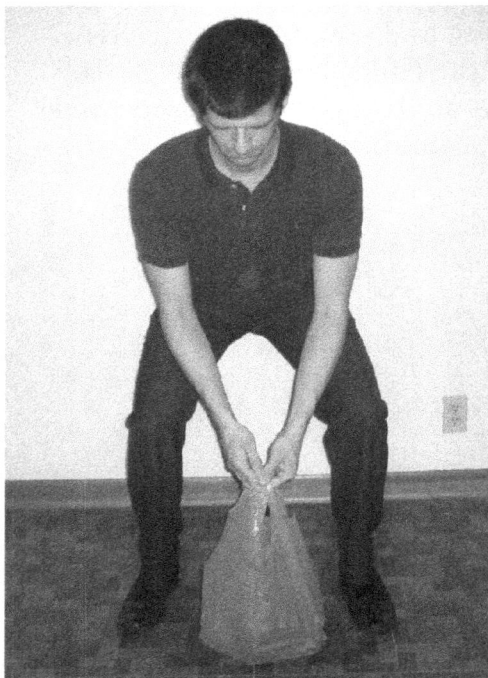

FIGURE 38 – GOOD   FIGURE 38A – BAD

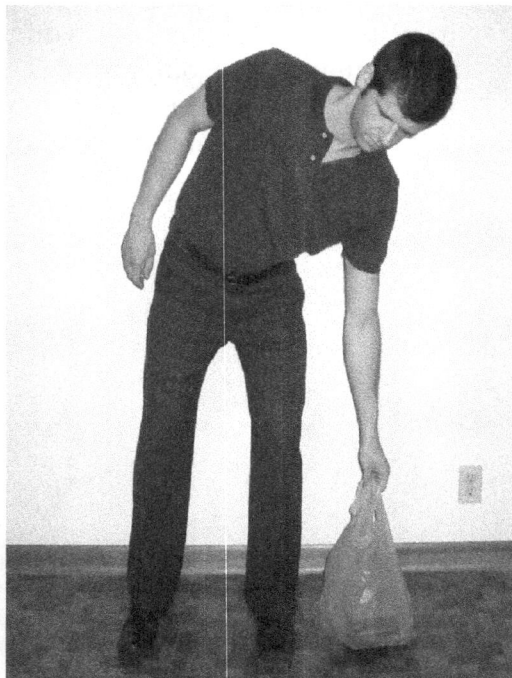

This advice applies primarily to bags with handles, which are typically used to transport groceries. The key to preventing back pain, when lifting a bag with handles, is to not shrug your shoulders and lean to one side when you pick up the bag (FIGURE 38A). If the bag is too heavy to pick up with your arm, squat and use your hand muscles to pick up the bag (2). Do not rely on your shoulder/neck muscles and low back to pick it up off the floor. An alternative is to squat down, pick up the bag with two hands and switch it to one hand (FIGURE 38).

RELATED NUMBERS: 1-2, 33-37

39. AVOID TWISTING TORQUE

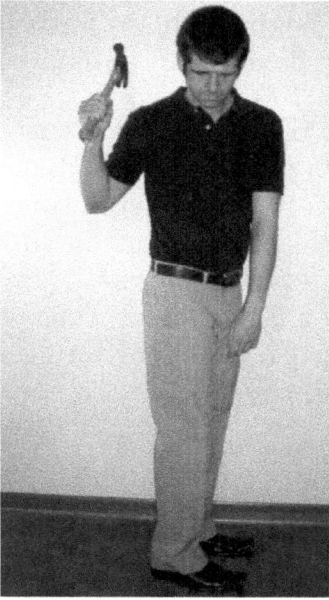
FIG.39 – BAD

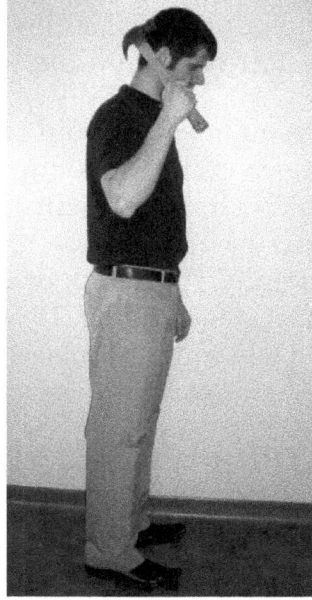
FIG.39A – GOOD

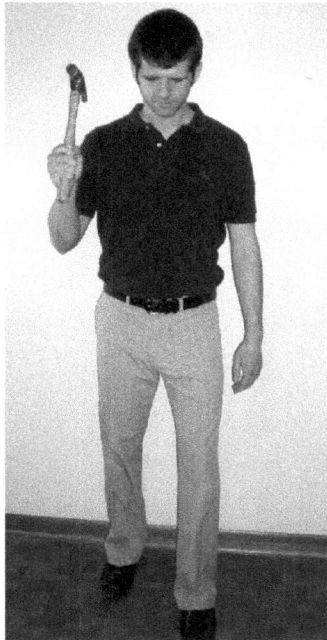
FIG.39B – GOOD

The simple act of twisting is not harmful to your body, unless it is immediately performed after you have fully flexed (bent) your spine. However, if you are a good reader, you would know to not ever fully flex your spine to begin with! As a result, do not fear twisting unless you just fully flexed your spine.

You need to avoid twisting torque (FIGURE 39). Twisting torque occurs when you rotate with a weight in your hand, for example, when you swing a sledgehammer or axe. Avoid this. Instead, use no rotation and swing the object over your head from behind your back or with your shoulder/arm alone (FIGURE 39A and B). If you must move a large object, turn your entire body and not just your torso. Do not rotate your torso, and you will not compromise the low back (4).

RELATED NUMBERS: 44, 47-48

40. PUSH AND PULL OBJECTS THROUGH YOUR LOW BACK

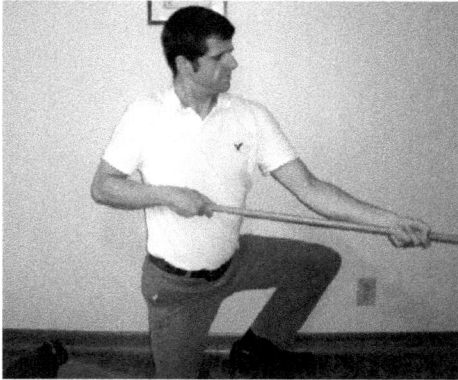

FIGURE 40 – GOOD

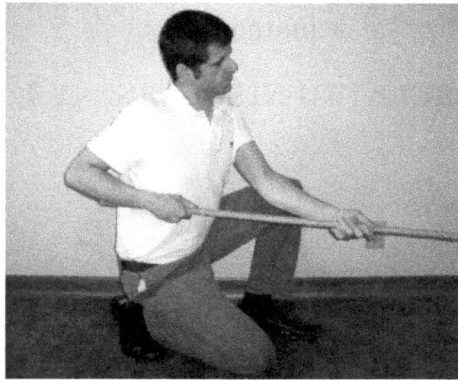

FIGURE 40A – GOOD

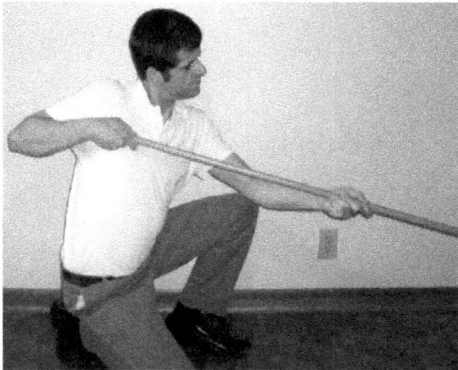

FIGURE 40B – BAD

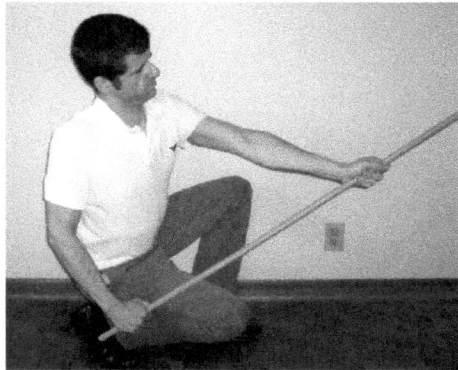

FIGURE 40C – BAD

The safest way to push or pull an object is to direct the force of the movement through your low back (FIGURE 40 and 40A). I will qualify the low back as the area between the bottom of your rib cage and the top of your hips. It is within this area that you should visualize a direct line of pull going into this region or out from the low back if you are pushing. In FIGURE 40B and 40C the force is not directed through the low back.

You may apply this same concept to opening doors. Each time you open a door, try to open the door with the force directed through the low back. People typically open doors with the force directed to the right or left of their body, which creates a twisting torque. Try directing the force of the door through your low back instead (4).

RELATED NUMBERS: 41-42,

41. PROPERLY PUSH A STROLLER/LAWNMOWER

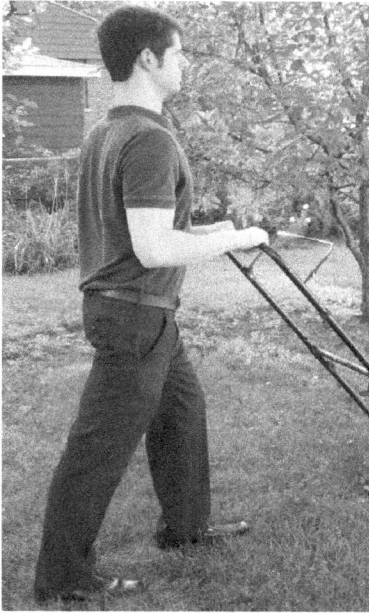

FIGURE 41 – GOOD

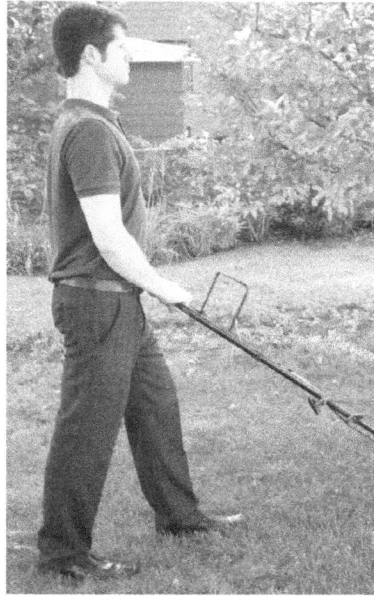

FIGURE 41A – BAD

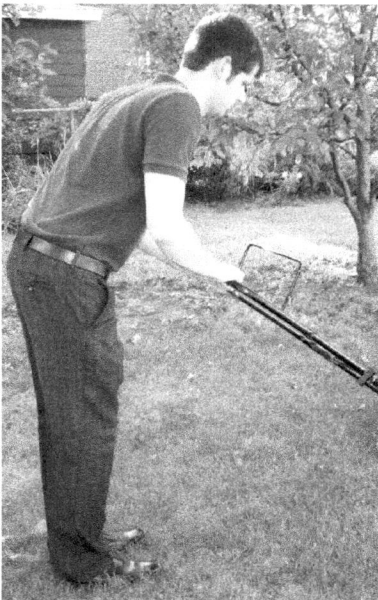

FIGURE 41B – BAD

The most important thing to consider when using a stroller or lawnmower is the height of the handles. When you push the stroller or lawnmower, the handles must be at a level that will prevent poor posture. If the handles are too low, it forces your back to bend forward, rounds your shoulders forward, and causes a forward head tilt (FIGURE 41B). Avoid this. Check the handle height and ensure you are not slouched while you push the object. Keep your spine neutral (straight) throughout the task. FIGURE 41A shows the force directed too far below the low back, which is wrong. Remember, the height of the handles should enable you to push the stroller/lawnmower with the force directed out of your low back, as in FIGURE 41 (2, 4).

RELATED NUMBERS: 1, 40, 42, 44

42. PROPERLY USE A WHEELBARROW

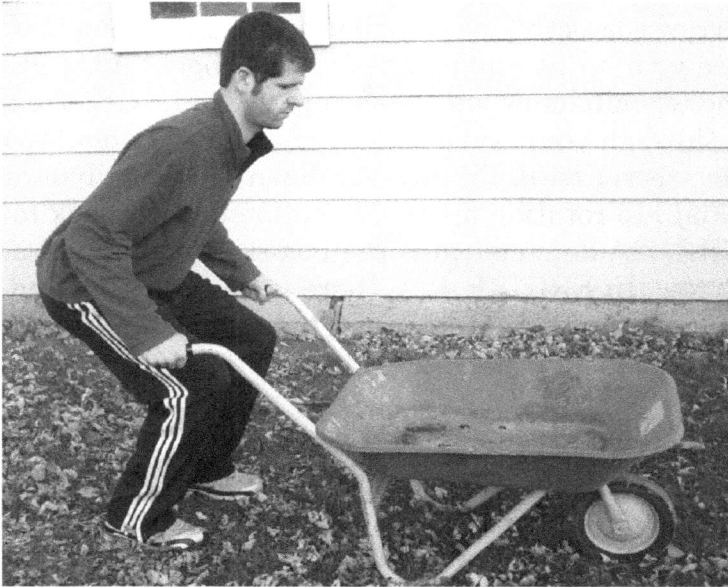

FIGURE 42 – GOOD

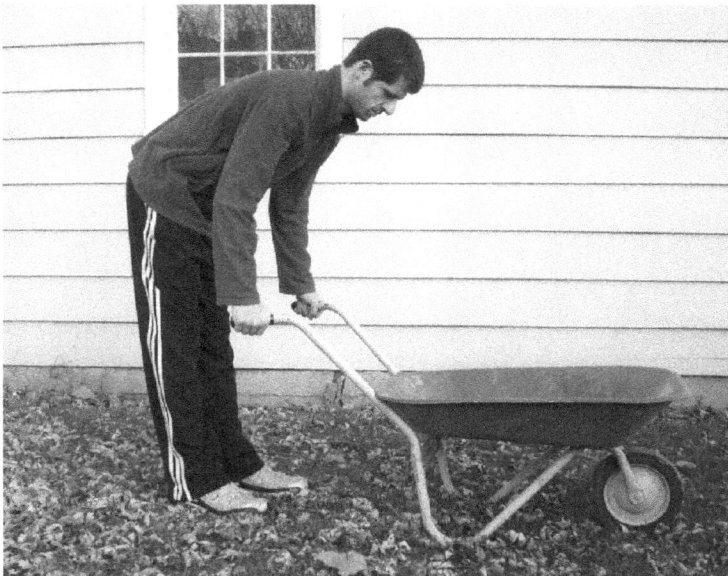

FIGURE 42A – BAD

There are several ways using a wheelbarrow can hurt your back. To prevent injury, make sure you lift the wheelbarrow correctly: use a squat and hip rotation (FIGURE 42). Spare your spine and do not flex your back! After properly lifting the wheelbarrow with your legs, push it with the force directed through your low back, as you would with a lawnmower or stroller (secret #40). Finally, set down the wheelbarrow using a squat and hip rotation again. Do not bend your back to lower it. FIGURE 42A demonstrates the incorrect way to use a wheelbarrow. In FIGURE 42A, there is no squatting and the back is flexed (bent). So, remember to bend your knees and rotate your hips.

RELATED NUMBERS: 1, 33-34, 40-41, 44

43. GARDEN PROPERLY

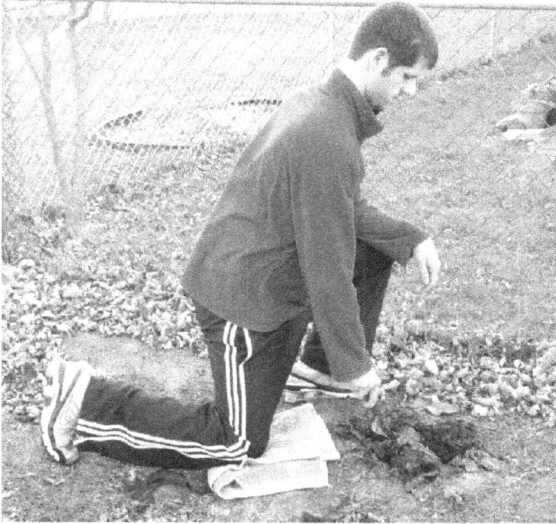

FIGURE 43 – GOOD

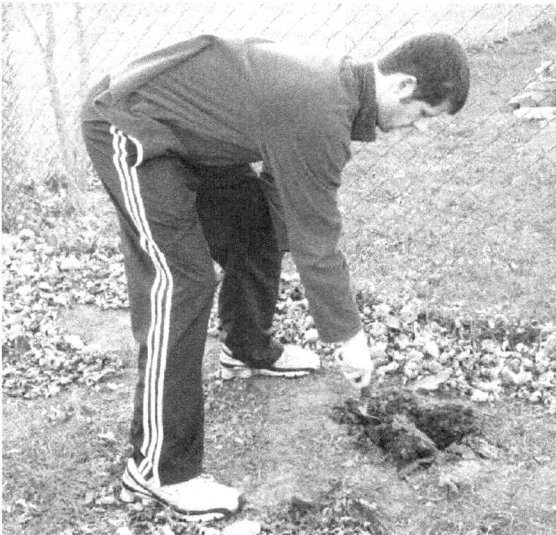

FIGURE 43A – BAD

People enjoy gardening, and for good reasons, too. Gardening is proven to have positive effects on its participants and may improve mental health (7)! It's a shame to think that gardening may cause your back pain, when it produces other positive benefits. Take these simple precautions to make sure gardening doesn't hurt your back. Don't bend down while you garden, as in FIGURE 43A. Instead, wear knee pads or kneel on a towel, or other padded item, to protect your knees. Kneel on one knee. Keep a neutral (straight) spine and use hip rotation (secret #33) to lean forward (FIGURE 43). Switch knees every few minutes or less depending on your comfort. There isn't a set rule for how long you should kneel before switching knees. It is based on comfort. It's important to remember not to flex your spine and to keep your back neutral (straight) while you garden.

RELATED NUMBERS: 1-2, 33

44. DIG/SHOVEL CORRECTLY

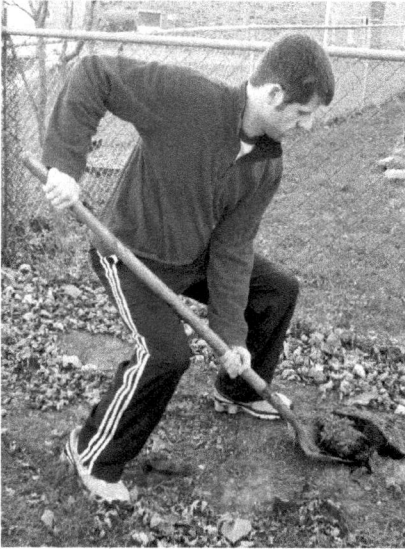

FIGURE 44 – GOOD

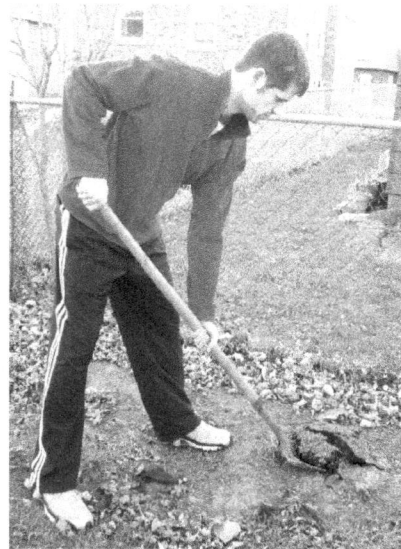

FIGURE 44A – BAD

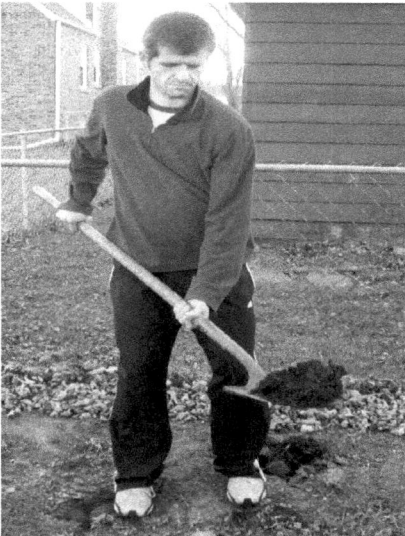

FIGURE 44B – GOOD

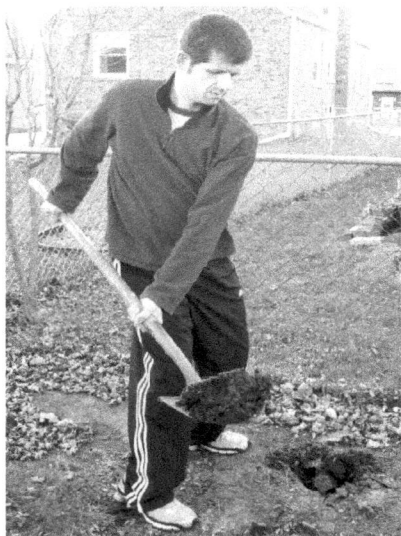

FIGURE 44C – BAD

Digging/shoveling isn't usually fun, but it becomes a real burden when it results in back pain. Although I can't make these tasks fun, I can reduce the risk of them hurting you. The number one thing to remember, when you're digging or shoveling, is to squat each time you perform the activity (FIGURE 44). Instead of bending your back to dig or shovel, squat. It's that easy. FIGURE 44A shows the incorrect way to dig. In FIGURE 44A, I am leaning over and stressing my back. After you squat, lift the load with your legs, not your back. Be certain you don't produce a twisting torque (secret #39), when you unload the dug/shoveled contents shown in FIGURE 44C. In FIGURE 44C, my feet are facing forward, but my body is twisted to the side. This is twisting torque. Instead, rotate your entire body (FIGURE 44B). Digging and shoveling should not cause you physical pain, if you avoid twisting and bending.

RELATED NUMBERS: 1, 34, 39-42

45. DO NOT BEND YOUR BACK LEANING OVER THE SINK

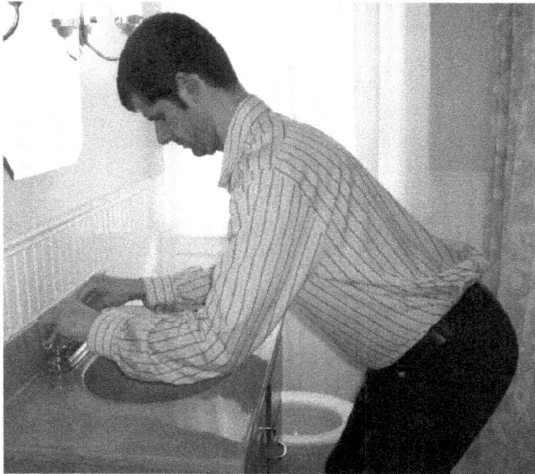

FIGURE 45 – GOOD

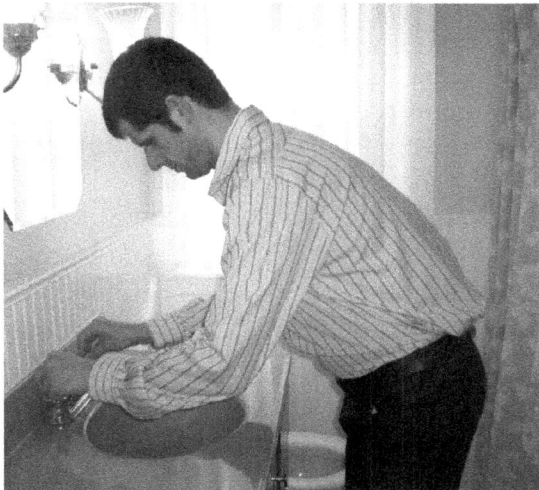

FIGURE 45A – BAD

People bend incorrectly over the sink to perform many tasks such as brushing their teeth, washing their face or hands, applying makeup, and removing contact lenses (FIGURE 45A). Instead of using your back to lean over the sink, squat and use hip rotation, as shown in FIGURE 45 (1, 2). Note in FIGURE 45A, the spine is flexed, whereas in FIGURE 45, the spine is spared using hip rotation.

RELATED NUMBERS: 1-2, 5, 33-34

46. CHANGE A BABY'S DIAPER PROPERLY

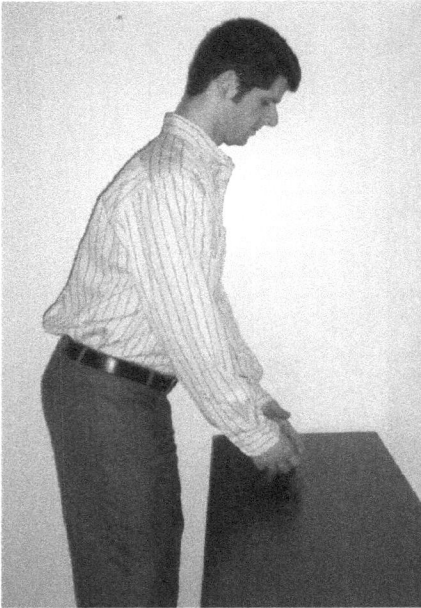

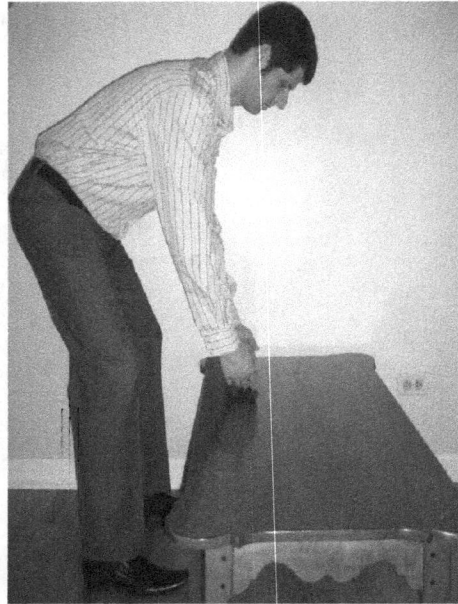

FIG.46 – GOOD   FIG.46A – BAD (C-SHAPE)

       Parents of newborns know too well how often a baby's diaper needs changing. Hopefully, you are not placing unnecessary stress on your back each time you perform this important task. Be sure to use a changing surface that is high enough to prevent flexion (bending) of the low back (FIGURE 46). Ideally, you want to select a changing station that prevents forward bending (2). However, if this is not feasible, use one of the back-sparing options to bend forward: squat or hip rotation. In FIGURE 46A, the changing surface is too low and the spine is flexed. Work at a proper height to protect your back.

RELATED NUMBERS: 1-2, 33-37

47. SWEEP PROPERLY

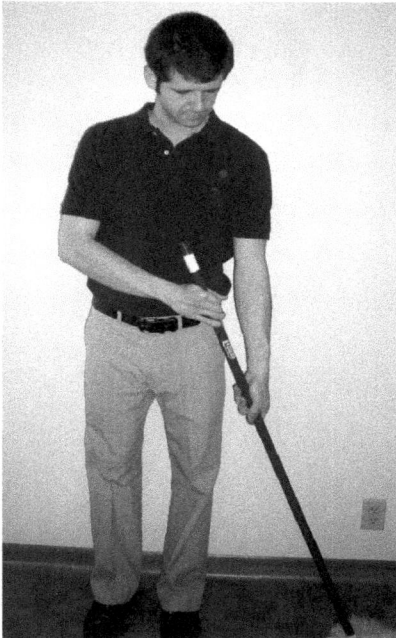

FIGURE 47 – GOOD

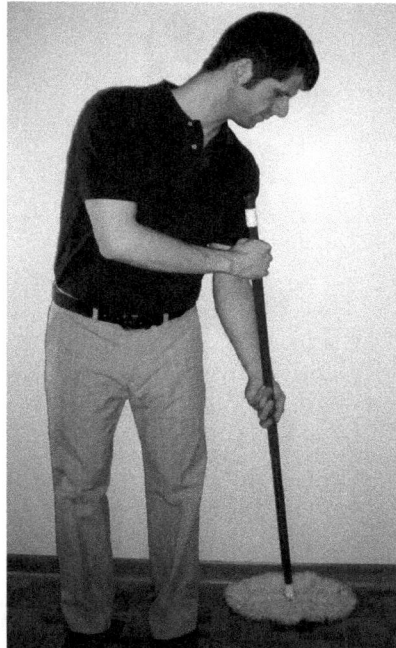

FIGURE 47A – BAD

Avoid twisting torque when sweeping with a broom or mop (FIGURE 47A). A broom is typically light-weight. However, twisting torque—or twisting with a weight in your hands—will likely cause back problems if done frequently, no matter the amount of weight. Let's play it safe. No twisting when you sweep. To properly sweep, hold the broom in front of you with two hands and sweep forward and backward. Another option is to hold the broom with two hands, but instead of sweeping forward and backward, use your arms to sweep from side to side (FIGURE 47). The idea is to avoid rotation (2).

RELATED NUMBERS: 1, 5, 39, 48

48. VACUUM CORRECTLY

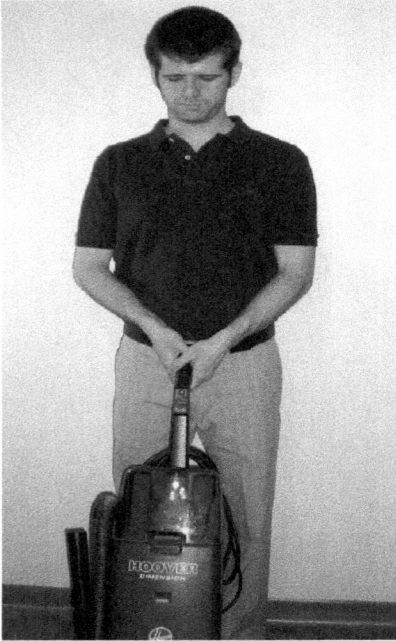

FIGURE 48 – GOOD

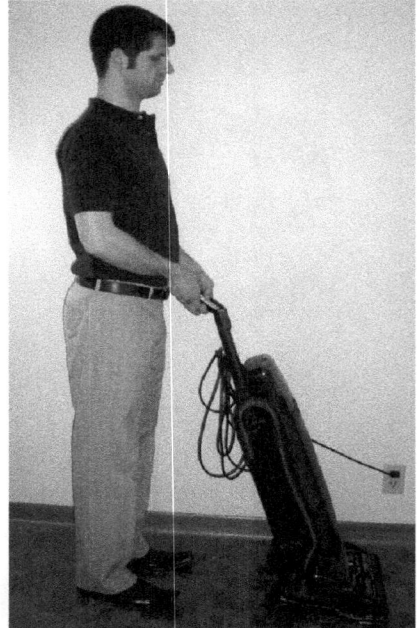

FIGURE 48A – GOOD

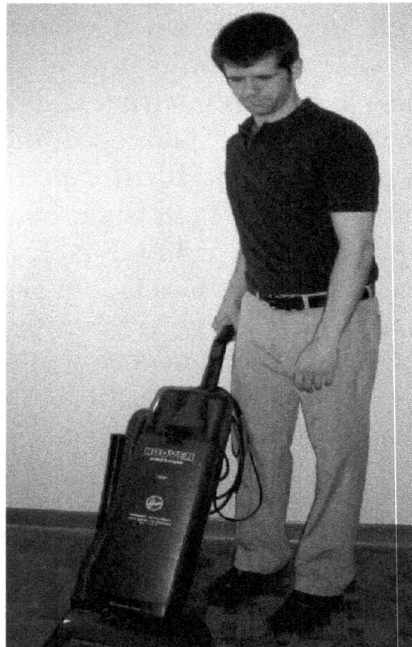

FIGURE 48B – BAD

In practice, patients complain that vacuuming is painful to them and they can't understand why. Vacuuming is painful when performed with a twisting torque, which stresses the low back (FIGURE 48B). The average person will not experience pain, but a patient with current back problems will notice discomfort immediately.

A common mistake while vacuuming is to hold the vacuum with one hand on either the right or left side of your body (FIGURE 48B). As mentioned, you must push or pull an object with the force directed through your low back in order to protect it (secret #40). Instead of using one hand to push the vacuum on either side of your body, hold the vacuum with two hands directly in front of you to ensure the force is directed through your low back as in FIGURE 48 and 48A (2, 4).

RELATED NUMBERS: 1, 5, 39, 40, 47

49. CARRY BACKPACK LOADS CORRECTLY

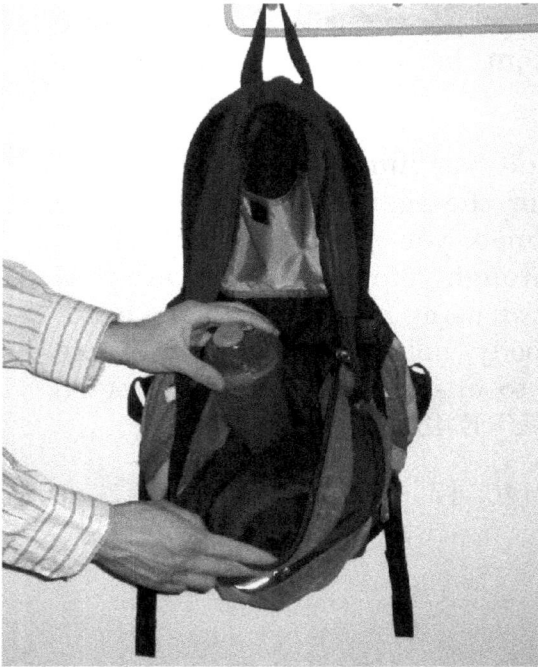

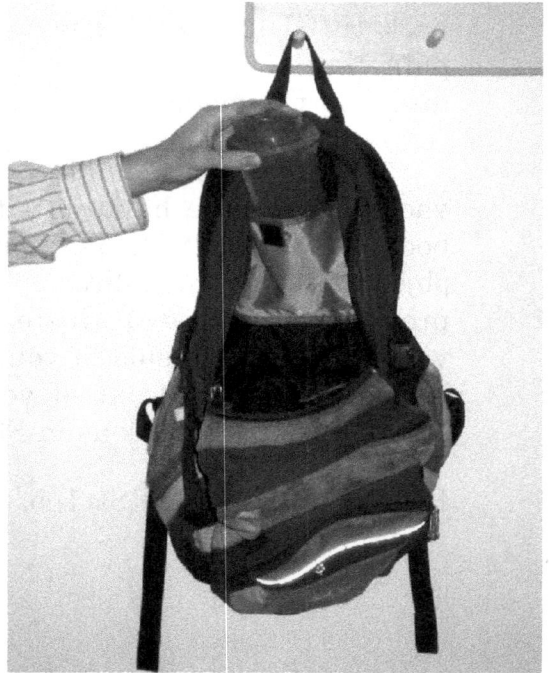

FIG.49 – ROUGH   FIG.49A – SMOOTH

Evidence shows that there is a particular way to carry objects in your backpack based on the environment in which you are walking. If you are walking through a rough, bumpy environment you should carry the load of your backpack at the very bottom of the pack (FIGURE 49). If you are walking over smooth ground, carry the load high in your pack (FIGURE 49A). The different walking environments produce varying stresses on the body. Placing the loads to accommodate the terrain can prevent back problems (4).

RELATED NUMBERS: 50

50. CARRY LESS THAN 10% OF YOUR BODY WEIGHT

People, specifically children, are likely to suffer from upper and mid back pain if they repeatedly carry greater than 10% of their body weight in backpacks over their shoulders. There is a correlation between backpack weight (greater than 10%) and an increase in missed school days. Children with back pain are more likely to develop back pain as an adult (3, 5). Luckily, there is an easy solution: keep less than 10% of your bodyweight in the backpack. I also recommend this rule for any bag worn over the shoulder, particularly women's purses!

RELATED NUMBERS: 49

51. BRING YOUR FEET UP TO YOU INSTEAD OF BENDING

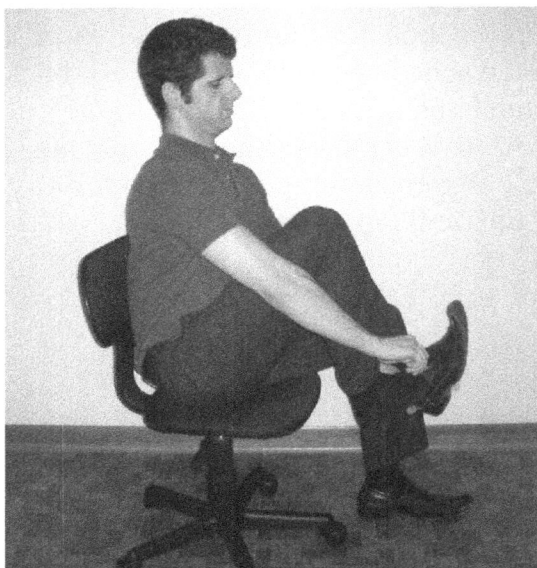

FIGURE 51 – GOOD

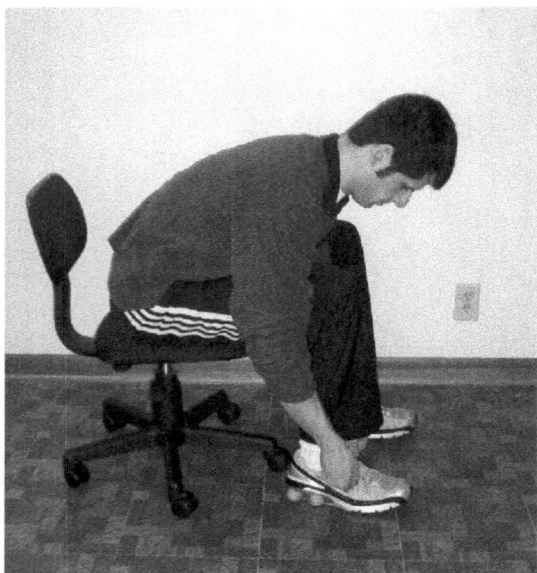

FIGURE 51A – BAD

This tactic applies when you are putting on your socks or shoes, cutting toenails, painting your nails, etc. Because of disc imbibition (secret #3), it is critical to raise your feet up to you instead of bending down, when you first awake (FIGURE 51). However, it is a good habit to use this technique all the time. Bringing your feet up to you instead of bending down to your feet will spare the back of full flexion and repetitive misuse (2). FIGURE 51A demonstrates the wrong way to perform this task. Bringing your feet up to you instead of bending down is an easy way to protect your back. You may also lay on your back in your bed and try bringing your feet up to you.

RELATED NUMBERS: 1-4

REFERENCES

1. Khalil, Tarek M., et al. *Ergonomics in Back Pain: A Guide to Prevention and Rehabilitation.* New York: Van Nostrand Reinhold, 1993. Print.
2. Liebenson, Craig. *Rehabilitation of the Spine: A Practitioners Manual.* 2nd ed. Baltimore: Lippincott, 2007. Print.
3. Mackenzie, W.G., et al. "Backpacks in Children." Clinical Orthopaedics and Related Research 409 (2003): 78-84. Print.
4. McGill, Stuart. *Low Back Disorders: Evidence-based Prevention and Rehabilitation.* 2nd ed. Champaign: Human Kinetics, 2007. Print.
5. Moore, M.J., et al. "Association of Relative Backpack Weight with Reported Pain, Pain Sites, Medical Utilization, and Lost School Time in Children and Adolescents." Journal of School Health 77.5 (2007): 232-39. Print.
6. Nordin, Margareta and Victor H. Frankel. *Basic Biomechanics of the Musculoskeletal System.* 3rd ed. Baltimore: Lippincott, 2001. Print.
7. Wakefield, S., et al. "Growing Urban Health: Community Gardening in South-East Toronto." Health Promotion International 2 (2007): 92-101. Print

CHAPTER 3: EXERCISES

DISCLAIMER:

The "EXERCISES" section is intended for those who are healthy enough to perform exercise. If you are unsure whether you are able to perform these exercises safely, please consult your physician. If you experience any pain during these exercises, stop, and consult your physician.

52. PERFORM BRIDGES

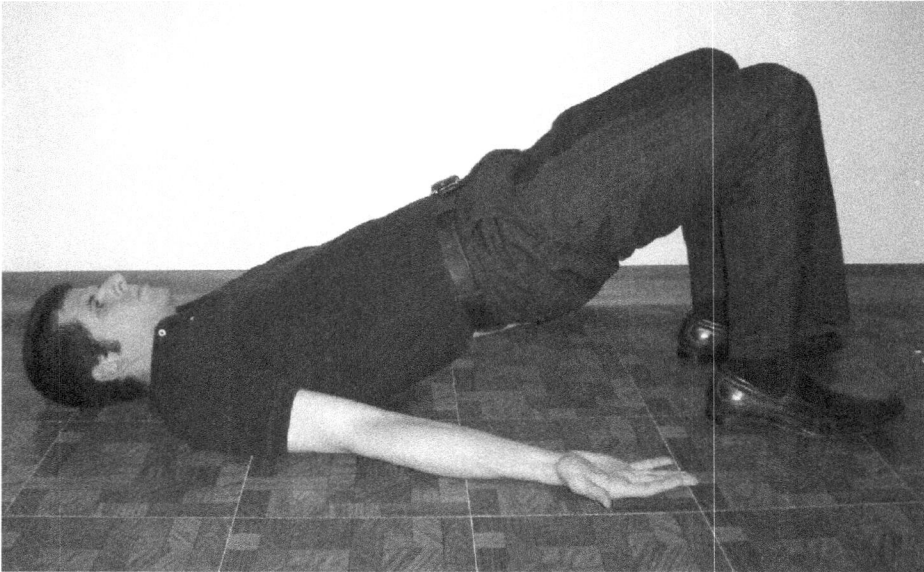

FIGURE 52 – SIMPLE BRIDGE

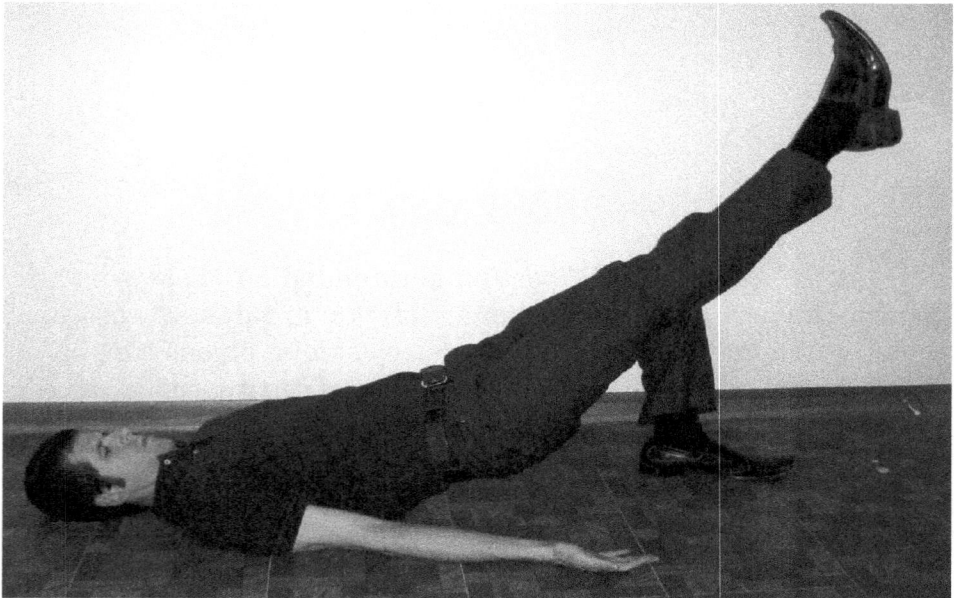

FIGURE 52A – ADVANCED BRIDGE

There is a correlation between back pain/injury and weak muscles known as the multifidus (small muscle in your back) and gluteus maximus, or glute (buttocks). You can strengthen these muscles with an exercise called the bridge. To perform the bridge, lay on your back with your knees bent and feet flat on the floor. Place your arms to the side of your torso with your hands, palms up, and fingers spread as widely as possible. Your feet should be shoulder-width apart and perpendicular to the ground. Next, contract your abdominal muscles and slowly bring your hips off the floor. Try to form a 45-degree angle between your body and the floor (FIGURE 52). Keep your spine neutral throughout the exercise. Hold this position for 3-5 seconds. Relax your stomach and lower your hips to the floor. Once your hips hit the floor, contract your stomach and bring your hips up again. Hold this position and repeat 8-10 times, if possible. Keep your hamstrings relaxed during this exercise, and contract your glutes. If you are contracting your hamstrings, you are performing the bridge incorrectly.

When you can perform the bridge 8-10 times as described, you may advance the exercise. To advance it, bring your hips off the floor and extend your left leg straight off the ground. Hold it extended for 1-2 seconds, lower it, and raise your right leg (FIGURE 52A). Again, keep it raised for 1-2 seconds. Lower your leg, relax your stomach and bring your hips down to the floor (1). Each time you raise your hips and extend both legs is one repetition. Repeat this exercise for 8-10 reps if possible. Increase the difficulty by increasing either the number of repetitions or the duration of time you hold your hips off the ground. Do not increase the number of repetitions and the duration.

RELATED NUMBERS: 53-55

53. PERFORM A SIDE BRIDGE

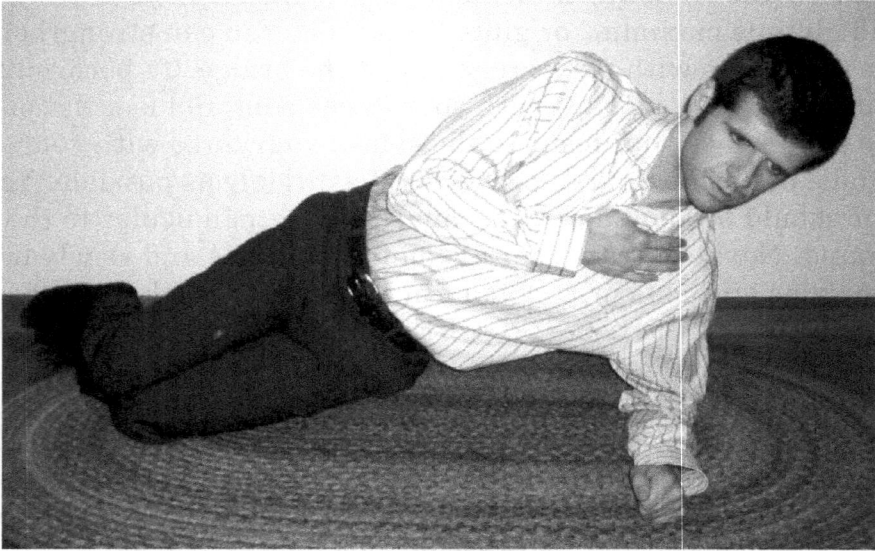

FIGURE 53 – SIMPLE SIDE BRIDGE

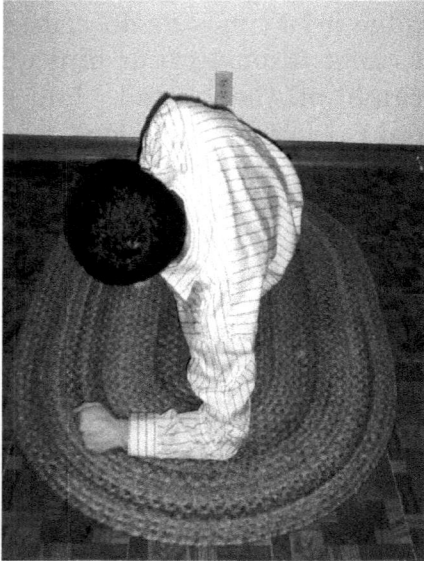

FIG.53A – ELBOW

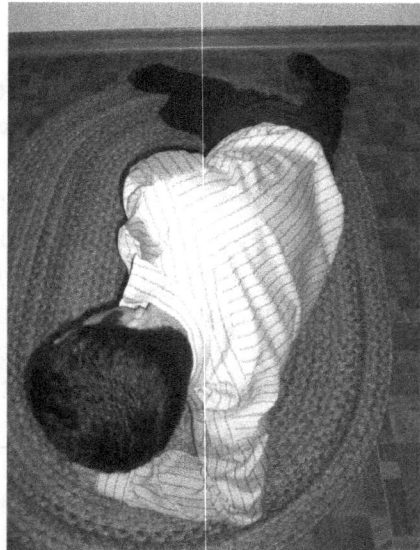

FIG.53B – IMAGINARY LINE

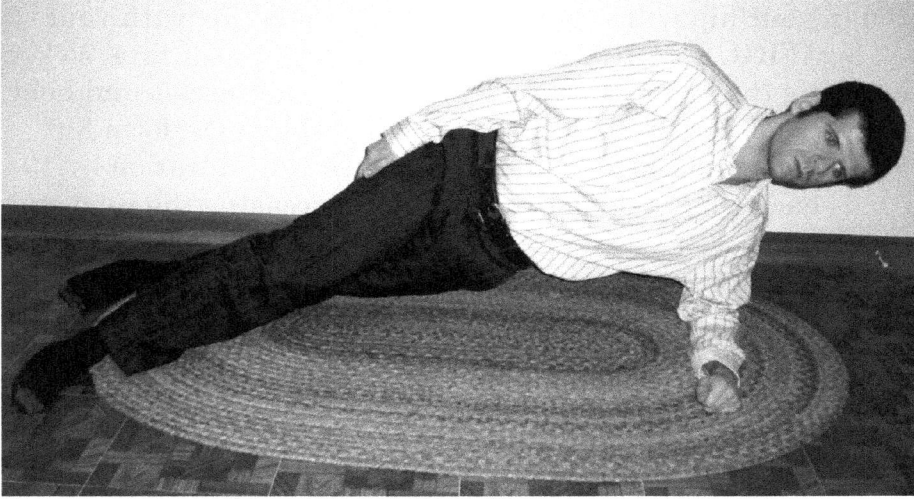

FIGURE 53C – ADVANCED SIDE BRIDGE

The quadratus lumborum (Q.L.) and transverse abdominus (Tr.A) are important stabilizing muscles of the spine. They are frequently neglected, but easy to strengthen. I believe the best exercise to strengthen the Q.L. and Tr.A is the side bridge, not to be confused with the bridge. As we discussed, the bridge is for strengthening the multifidi and glutes. As the name implies, the side bridge is performed by lying on your side. Once on your side, bend your knees to 90 degrees. Next, use your elbow to support your torso's body weight. Keep your elbow perpendicular to the floor, and your shoulder should form a straight line with your hips and thighs (FIGURE 53A and 53B). Contract your abdominal muscles. Finally, raise your hips off the ground so that your body forms a 45 degree angle with the floor. Your hips and elbow support your body weight. You may place your free hand on your opposite shoulder to increase the difficulty (FIGURE 53). Try to hold this position for 10 seconds and relax. This is one rep. Do 3-5 reps. When you can perform 3-5 reps at 30 seconds each, you are ready to advance.

The advanced bridge involves straightening your legs and using your feet and elbow to support your body weight. Your feet should not be on top of each other. Your top leg should move forward and your back leg moves behind you (FIGURE 53C) (3).

The imaginary straight line coming from your shoulder and through your hip will continue down to form a line with your back leg (FIGURE 53B). It is the same concept as before, so keep everything the same. Contract your stomach muscles and hold for 10 seconds. Do 3-5 reps. Once you are able to perform 3-5 reps at 30 seconds each, you may increase your duration by 10 seconds each time. I do not recommend increasing the reps and duration.

RELATED NUMBERS: 52, 54-55

54. PERFORM PLANKS

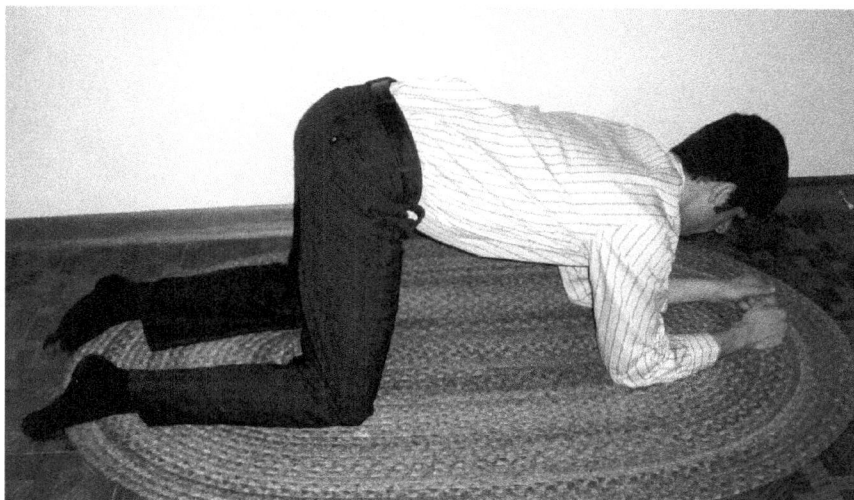

FIGURE 54 – STARTING POSITION

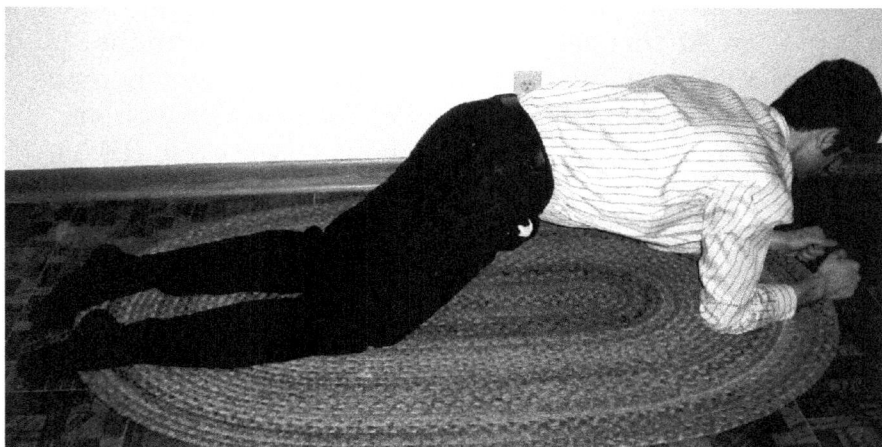

FIGURE 54A – MOVING YOUR KNEES

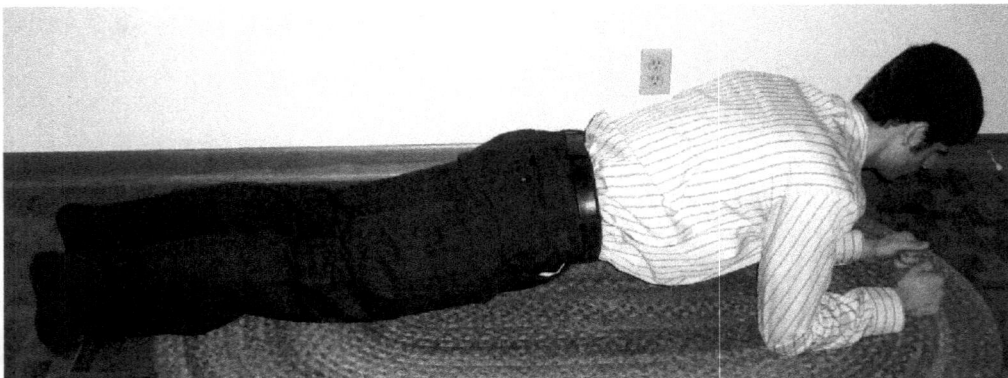

FIGURE 54B – ADVANCED PLANK

Another exercise to strengthen the spine stabilizing muscles is the plank. The plank targets the transverse abdominus, quadratus lumborum, and abdominals. To perform a plank, support your body with your forearms and knees, which are shoulder-width apart. Instead of supporting your body weight with your hands, you are using your forearms. Be sure to have the palm side of your hands facing each other, as you form them into fists. At this point, your upper arms and thighs should be perpendicular to the floor (FIGURE 54). Next, slowly move your knees further away from your forearms so that you are beginning to support your body with your torso (FIGURE 54A). Once it becomes difficult to hold this position and you feel tension in your stomach, stop moving your knees. Contract your stomach muscles, as if you are bracing for a punch to the gut, and try to hold that position for 10 seconds. Do this 3-5 times at 10 seconds each.

As this becomes easier, move your knees further away from your last hold position and repeat. Contract your stomach muscles each time. Eventually, the goal is to support your body weight with your forearms and toes. The advanced form of this exercise uses your feet and forearms to hold your body weight, as shown in FIGURE 54B (3). Try to work towards 3-5 repetitions at 60 seconds each in the advanced position. If you can achieve this, your spine will have steel beams of muscle reinforcing it!

RELATED NUMBERS: 52-53, 55

55. AVOID PRONE BACK EXTENSIONS

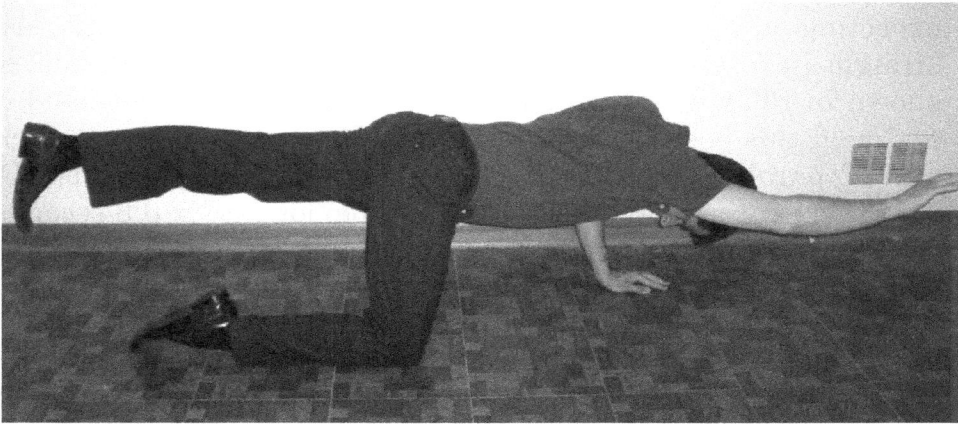

FIGURE 55 – GOOD

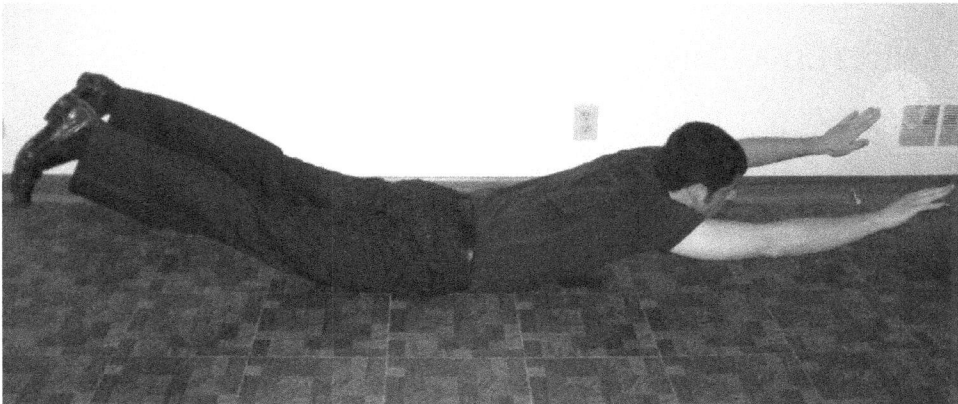

FIGURE 55A – BAD

A common exercise is the prone back extension (FIGURE 55A). This exercise does a great job of activating certain back muscles, but it also does a great job of placing large amounts of stress on your low back. The prone back extension places 6,000 Newtons (Newtons, abbreviated "N," is a measurement of force.) on the back. You should avoid this exercise (4).

It is important to strengthen these muscles in your back. A safer exercise is a bird-dog (FIGURE 55). To perform the bird-dog, start on your hands and knees. Place your hands and knees at 90 degrees, so that your arms and thighs are perpendicular to the floor. Contract your stomach muscles, as if you were expecting a punch in the stomach. Extend your right arm straight in front of you and your left leg straight behind you, as shown in FIGURE 55. Keep your spine neutral—do not bend it, and hold this position for 6-8 seconds. Be sure to keep your arm and leg parallel with the ground, as you perform the exercise. Do not raise your arm and leg too high or too low. After 6-8 seconds, rest your arm and leg and perform the exercise with your opposite side. Again, hold your leg and arm extended for 6-8 seconds (3). Performing this exercise with both arms and legs constitutes one rep. Do 8-10 reps. Once you are able to hold the position for 6-8 seconds for 8 reps, move on to 9 and 10 reps. If you complete 10 reps at 8 seconds each, try holding the position for 10-12 seconds. Increase the duration of each set to increase the difficulty.

RELATED NUMBERS: 52-54

56. PERFORM SIT-UPS CORRECTLY

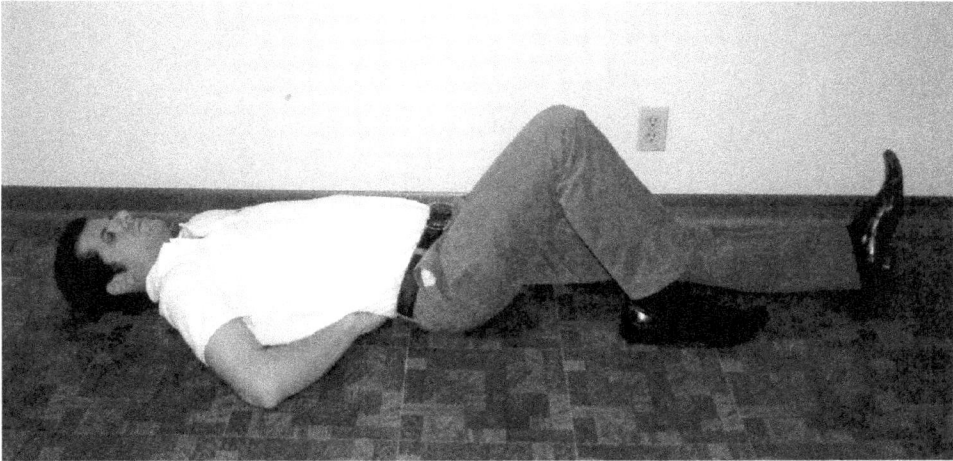

FIGURE 56 – STARTING POSITION

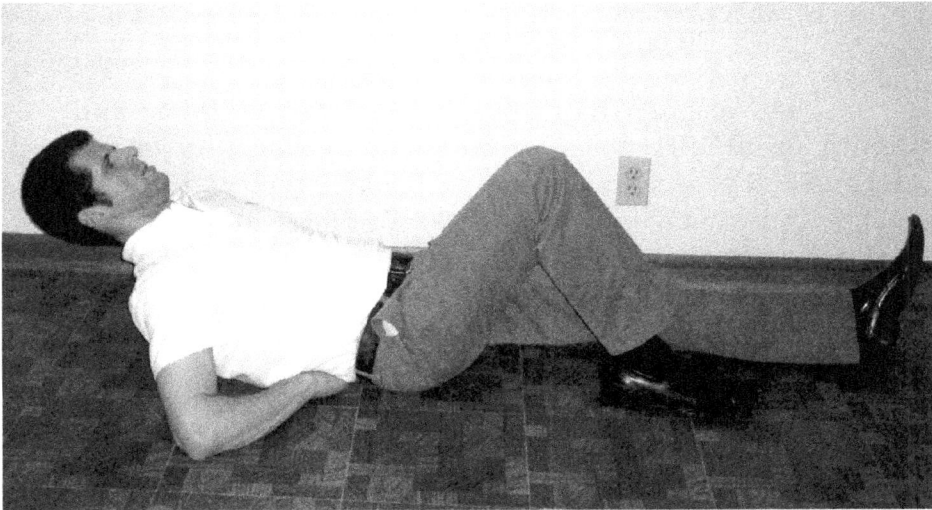

FIGURE 56A – END POSITION

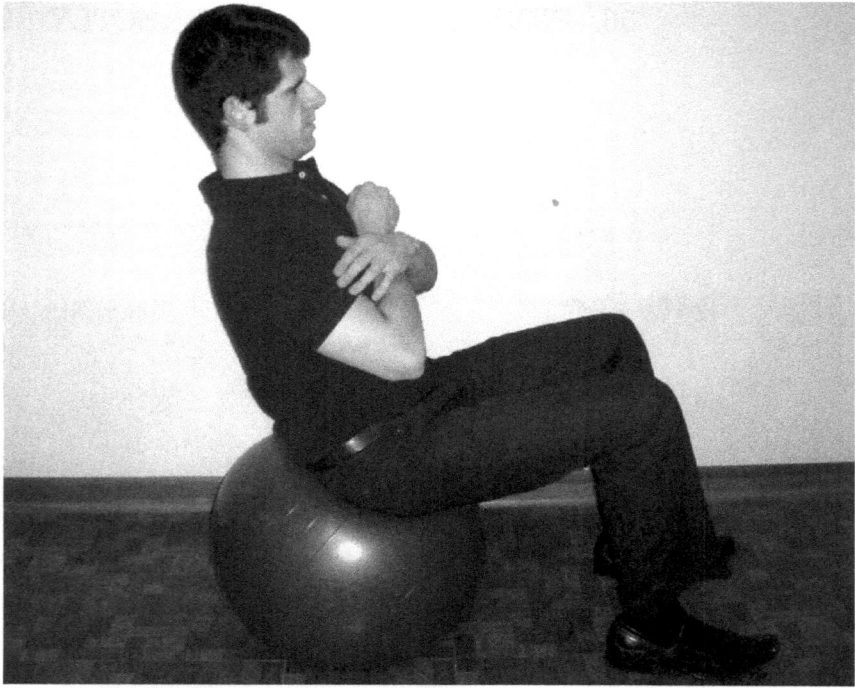

FIGURE 56B – GOOD

The National Institute for Occupational Safety and Health, or NIOSH, doesn't recommend performing job tasks that exceed 3300 N of force on the low back. A typical sit-up (lying on back with knees bent) places 3300 N of force on the low back each time one is performed. Tasks that exceed 3300 N of force are linked to a higher likelihood of back injuries. You should avoid activities that place your back at risk, yet you are likely performing a sit-up incorrectly each day.

A safer way to perform sit-ups is to lie on your back, with your hands placed palm down underneath the low back. Your low back should not be flush with the ground. There should be an "inverted C-shape" curve in your low back for your hands to fit underneath it. Bend one leg (FIGURE 56). It can be either your left or right, as it doesn't matter. Keep your head and torso in the same plane as you flex your torso to 45 degrees (FIGURE 56A). This method is the proper way to perform a sit-up without injury. Performing a sit-up in the manner described above places approximately 2000 N of force on the low back compared to the 3300 N of force generated by the typical sit-up (3).

I also recommend sitting on an exercise ball, as an alternative method (FIGURE 56B), to perform a sit-up if you aren't able to lie on your back as described above. Performing sit-ups on an exercise ball reduces the amount of force on your back as well (4). If you perform a sit-up on an exercise ball, keep your back neutral (straight) and do not come up higher than 90 degrees.

RELATED NUMBERS: 1-2

57. DO NOT FLEX/HYPEREXTEND YOUR BACK PERFORMING DEADLIFTS

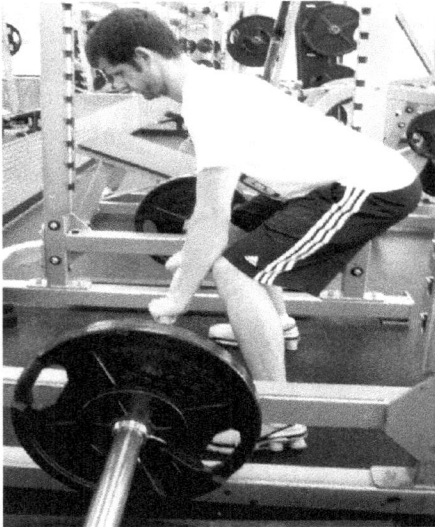

FIGURE 57 – GOOD

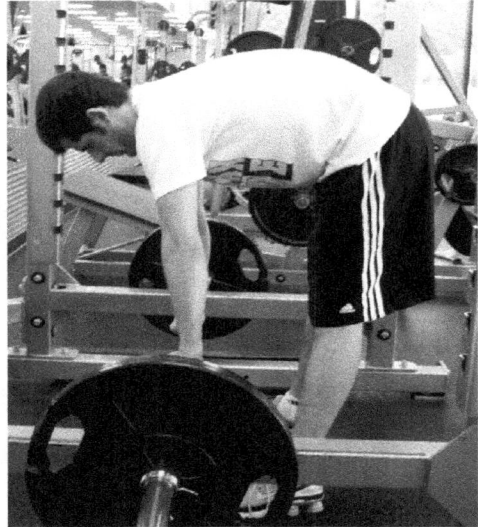

FIGURE 57A – BAD

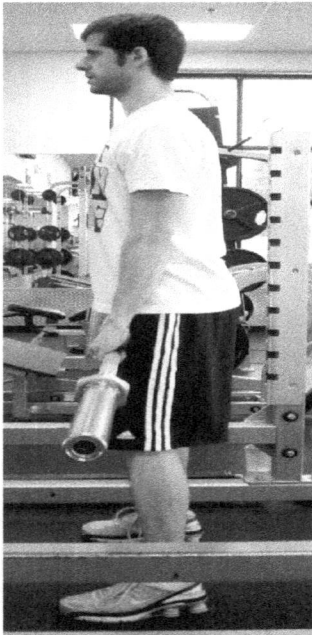

FIGURE 57B – GOOD

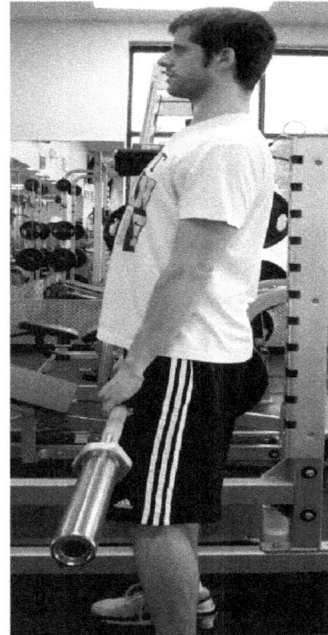

FIGURE 57C – BAD

A common body-building exercise is the deadlift. The deadlift strengthens the paraspinal muscles, or the extensors, of the mid-back. The key to not hurting your low back during this exercise is to remember hip rotation (FIGURE 57). Do NOT flex/bend your back while executing the deadlift (FIGURE 57A). The important things to remember when performing hip rotation is to first to stick out your butt. Next, keep your back neutral (straight) and the weight as close to your body as possible. From there, rotate your hips with a neutral back, as you lift the weight. Be certain NOT to extend your back past 180 degrees (FIGURE 57C). Extending too far backward irritates your low back joints (2, 3). Keep your back perfectly straight, or perpendicular to ground, as you reach the end of your lift (FIGURE 57B) to decrease your risk of injury.

RELATED NUMBERS: 1-2, 33-34

58. SWING YOUR GOLF CLUB CORRECTLY

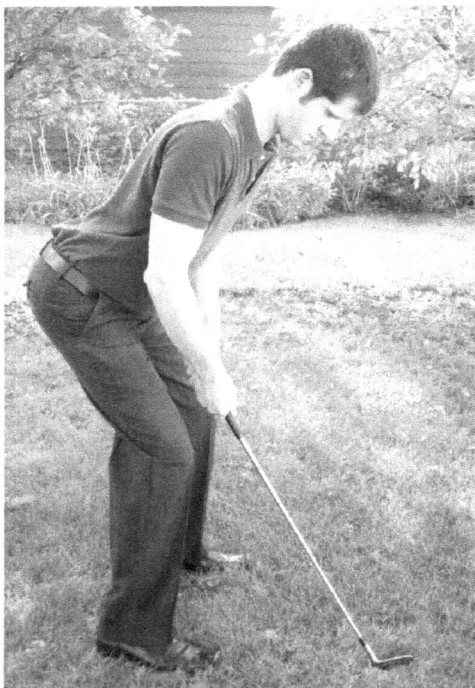

FIGURE 58 – GOOD   FIGURE 58A – BAD

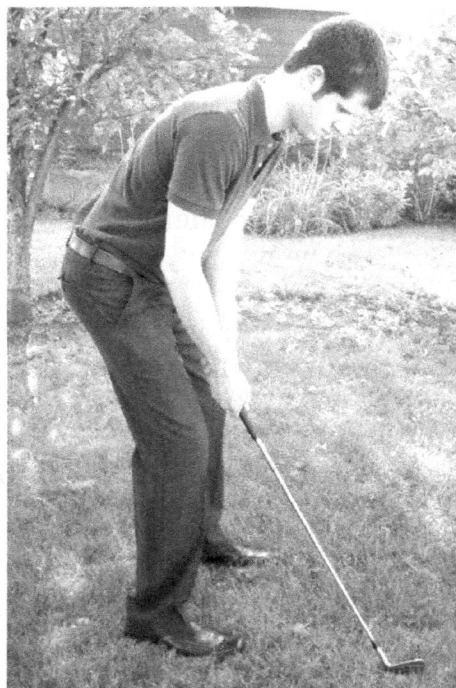

Relax, golfers, you don't have to change your swing—just your stance. Instead of using your back to bend forward as you prepare to swing (FIGURE 58A), use hip rotation to get your body in the forward golfing stance (FIGURE 58). Continue with your normal swing from here. This applies to driving the ball, chipping, and putting. Don't flex your back, rotate with your hips. See "hip rotation" (secret #33) to review the proper way to perform this procedure. Remember, you don't want to flex your back in any activity (2, 3).

RELATED NUMBERS: 1-2, 33-35

59. PERFORM A DYNAMIC STRETCH INSTEAD OF A STATIC STRETCH

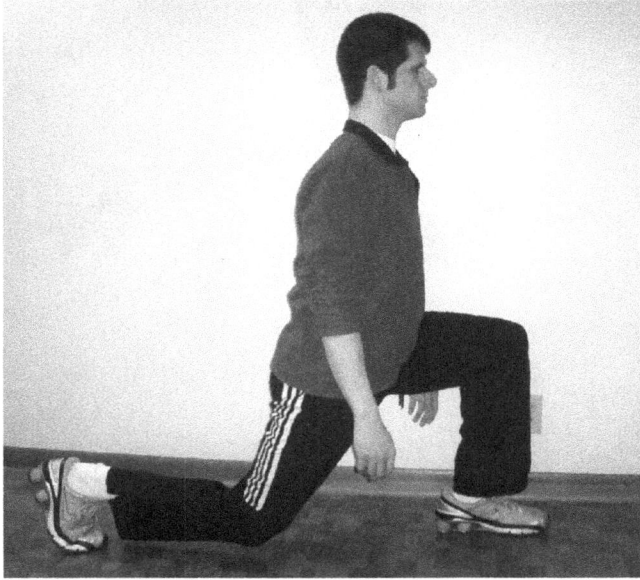

FIGURE 59 – DYNAMIC STRETCH

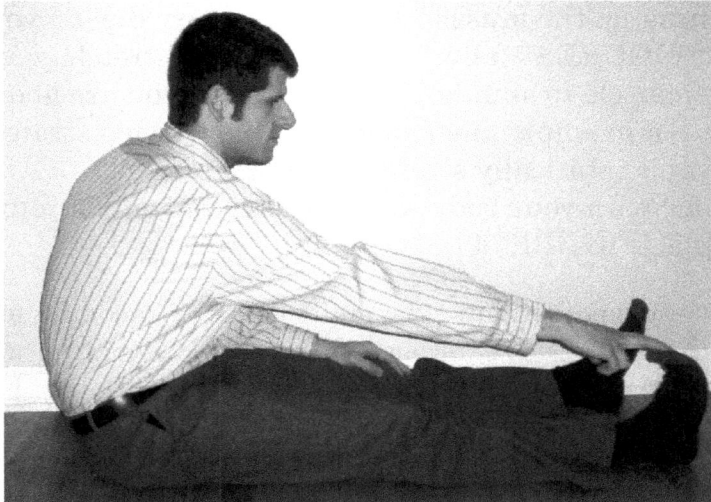

FIGURE 59A – STATIC STRETCH

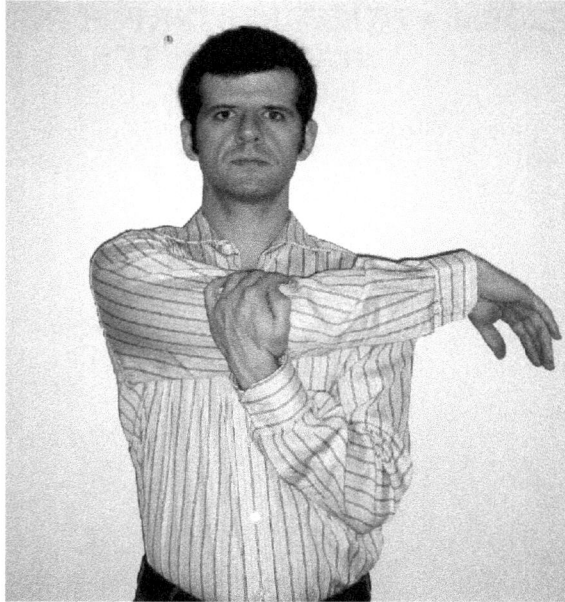

FIGURE 59B – STATIC STRETCH

Performing a dynamic stretch as a pre-workout warm-up is more effective in preventing injury than a static stretch (2). A static stretch is the "typical" stretch. In a static stretch, you hold a muscle in a position for an extended amount of time in hopes of "loosening up the muscle" to prevent injury during your workout (FIGURES 59A & B). In a dynamic stretch, you actively move the muscle to simulate the exercise(s) you are about to perform. For example, instead of holding your leg straight out in front of you to statically stretch your hamstrings (FIGURE 59A), use a lunge with your body weight to dynamically stretch your hamstrings (FIGURE 59).

As a rule of thumb for weight-lifting, I recommend performing the actual exercise as a dynamic warm-up with about 50% less weight instead of statically stretching. For example, before bench pressing, I recommend doing the bench press with 50% less weight for 10-12 reps than you would use for your actual exercise. Do this instead of a static stretch, which may involve holding your arm in a prolonged position prior to benching (FIGURE 59B).

60. AVOID THE ANGLED SQUAT MACHINE

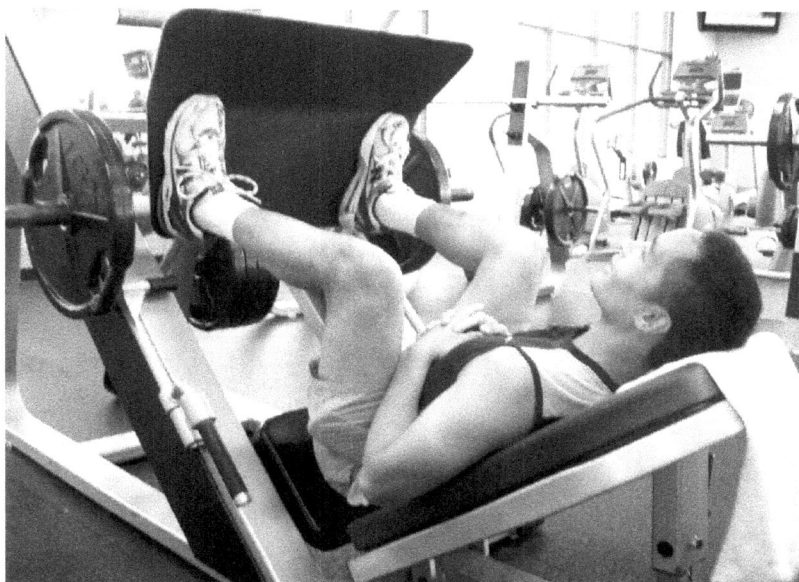

FIGURE 60 – AVOID THIS

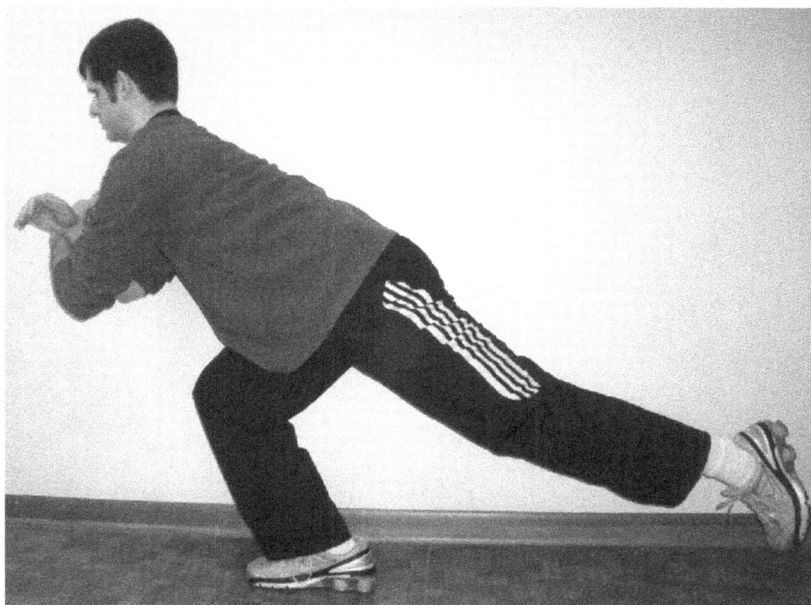

FIGURE 60A – GOOD

I do not recommend using the angled squat machine (FIGURE 60) as you are more likely to place your back in a flexed-position during the exercise, which you want to avoid. A flexed spine is 20-40% weaker than a neutral spine and more susceptible to injury (3). A seated leg curl-up machine is better. However, I recommend using single-leg squats to strengthen the quads, as they are the most functional (FIGURE 60A).

When you perform a single-leg squat, don't bend your knee past 90 degrees. Keep your back straight (neutral), not flexed. If you are able to perform three sets of 6-8 reps with your body weight, hold a five pound weight in your hand to increase the weight and difficulty. Increase the weight by five pounds as needed.

RELATED NUMBERS: 1-2

REFERENCES

1. Hyde, Thomas E., and Marianne S. Gengenbach. *Conservative Management of Sports Injuries.* 2nd ed. Boston: Jones, 2007. Print.
2. Liebenson, Craig. *Rehabilitation of the Spine: A Practitioners Manual.* 2nd ed. Baltimore: Lippincott, 2007. Print.
3. McGill, Stuart. *Low Back Disorders: Evidence-based Prevention and Rehabilitation.* 2nd ed. Champaign: Human Kinetics, 2007. Print.
4. Nordin, Margareta, and Victor H. Frankel. *Basic Biomechanics of the Musculoskeletal System.* 3rd ed. Baltimore: Lippincott, 2001. Print.

ACKNOWLEDGEMENTS

I could not have written this book without the unwitting help of the countless patients I encountered that wanted to get better. It was only through these patients' inquisitive minds and zeal to find the cause of their problems that enabled me to write this book. I learned that, if given the option, most people truly would prefer to find the cause of their injuries and not just take a pill to mask their symptoms.

I thank Mike Gilmartin for providing me with some amazingly kind words and insight. He probably didn't realize it, but Mike inspired me and everyone around him as we witnessed him successfully balance personal health with professional expectations. Mike also suggested that I contact Dr. Mark Hutchinson for which I'm grateful.

I also thank Dr. Mark Hutchinson for his constructive criticism, meaningful suggestions, and willingness to help a young chiropractor take his vision to the next step. Dr. Hutchinson's validation of my work was a big moment for me.

Thanks to Jamie Haro and Dana Cavalea:

Jamie—I appreciated your perseverance and devotion to helping me acquire one of the last pieces of my puzzle. Nothing is stronger than the bond of a Warrior, and you proved that convincingly. Ring out ahoya!

Dana—I never thought I'd like anything about a New York baseball team, but you proved me wrong. Despite your exhausting schedule and chaotic life, you still found time to read over my work and compliment it perfectly. Thanks.

Dr. George Goodman, despite running a first-rate institution, made the time to read my manuscript and respond in a timely fashion. Dr. Goodman also presented me with humbling compliments and encouragement. Thank you.

Trevor and Maria Gilbert supplied the best photographs in the entire book. The pictures turned out great, and Reese is a star!

You two gave my readers a chance to not have to look at me for once. My readers and I thank you.

Another thank you goes to Eric Dangoy, who contributed the best illustration of my book and another opportunity for my readers to look at someone else. If the police gig doesn't work out, rest assured you can find work as an illustrator.

And last, but hardly least, I owe an enormous thank you to my parents. Their editing, critiques, and recommendations made this book what it is, but it's their encouragement that made this book possible.

Note: Numbers here refer to pages, not "secrets" or safety tips.

INDEX

INDEX (CONT.)

ABOUT THE AUTHOR

Dr. Zumstein is a graduate of Marquette University and Logan College of Chiropractic. He is a doctor of chiropractic, owns a master's degree in sports rehab and science, and is certified in acupuncture and applied kinesiology. He has worked with and treated Division I collegiate and professional athletes.

Dr. Zumstein is the founder of The Back Safety and Wellness Consultants, which is dedicated to educating the public on preventing, reducing, and eliminating back and neck pain. You can learn more about The Back Safety and Wellness Consultants at www.backsafetyandwellness.com. Dr. Zumstein currently resides outside Chicago, where he practices chiropractic and consulting part-time.

Dr. Zumstein enjoys spending time with his family, reading, working out, following most Chicago sports teams, and playing his guitar.

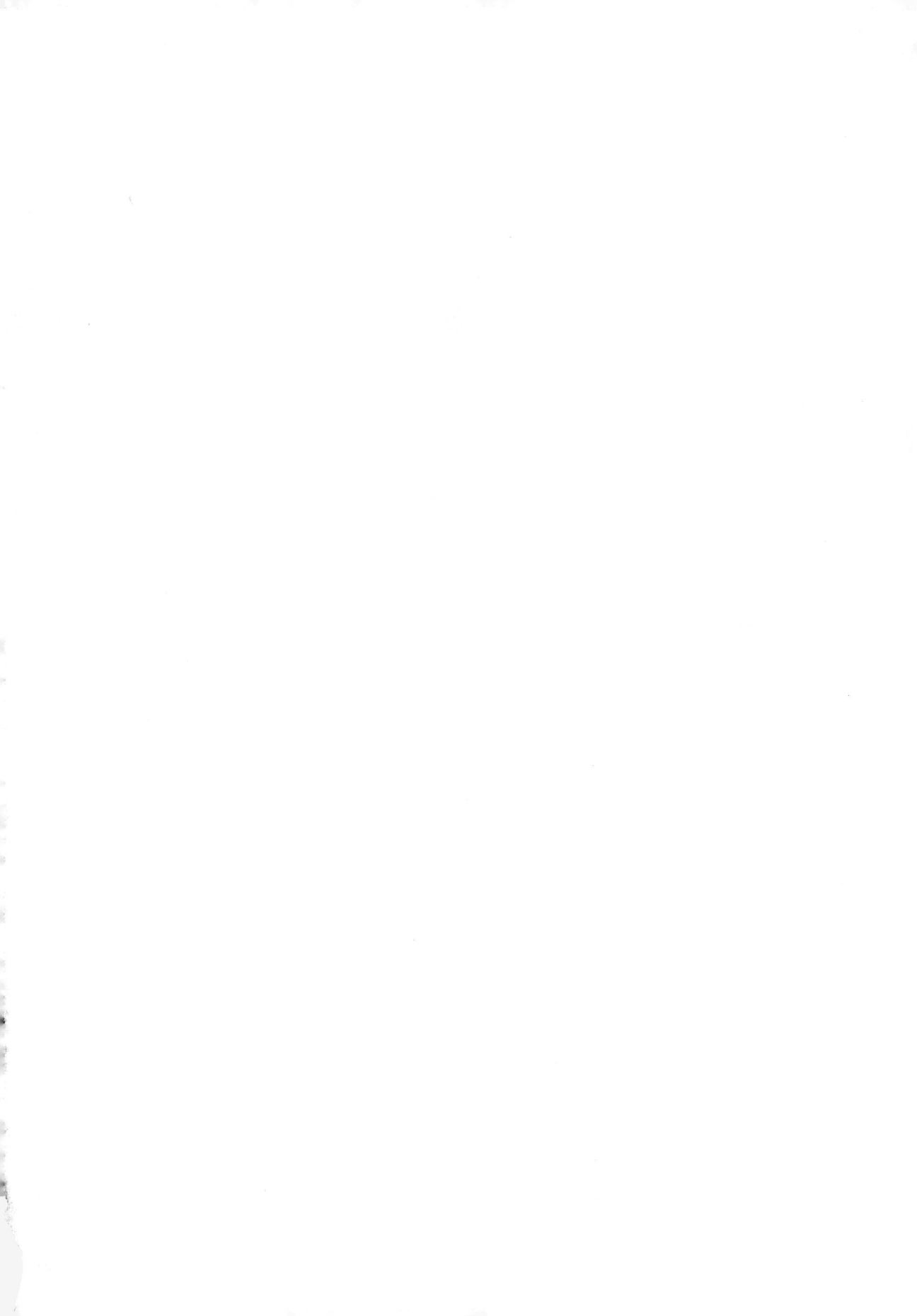